"This is an incredibly important book for group therapists working in an environment, impacted today by the psychology of polarisation, discrimination, and dehumanization. Dr. Abernethy has assembled an outstanding cadre of group therapy experts reflecting unparalleled breadth and depth of expertise. They each write in ways that are scholarly and accessible as they address racial dynamics, racism, identity dynamics, and internalised beliefs about race, privilege, and power. This text illustrates powerfully the theory, principles and practices group leaders require to understand, recognise, and work constructively as well as courageously in their groups."

Molyn Leszcz, *MD, FRCPC, CGP, AGPA-DF,*
professor of psychiatry, University of Toronto, past-president,
the American Group Psychotherapy Association

"Abernethy and colleagues have curated a compelling volume of pertinent and vital, culturally sensitive group therapy practices, that integrates diversity and a multiculturally oriented frame into the core of ethical and attuned clinical work. The authors provide clear ideas and direction that will guide the group therapy practitioner into a more systems-informed framework, that invites attention to power and dominance and how the need to dismantle dominance is just as foundational to our work as symptom reduction and healing. A must read for anyone wanting to expand and enhance their multiculturally informed teaching and practice as a justice oriented and thoughtful group psychotherapist."

Michele D. Ribeiro, *EdD, ABPP, CGP; (co) editor of The College Counselor's*
Guide to Group Psychotherapy and Examining Social Identities and
Diversity Issues in Group: Knocking at the Boundaries

"This book is a compass for navigating the intricate terrain of diversity dynamics encountered within group therapy. Through a diverse tapestry of authorial voices and perspectives, the book weaves in various theoretical frames from mindfulness, systems-centered, to MCO with case examples and visual metaphors to aid the reader in illuminating their own diversity consciousness. From exploring unique intersectional identities to reflections on systemic training practices, each chapter provides a unique fruit that is a joy to taste and explore with accessible case studies and frameworks, making it an indispensable resource and a step towards weaving diversity consciousness into the fabric of group therapy practice."

Vinny Malik Dehili, *Ph.D, ABPP, CGP, Board Certified in Group Psychology,*
co-chair, Diversity, Equity, & Inclusion Taskforce, American Group
Psychological Association, program chair American Psychological
Association Division 49 (Group Psychology), vice president of
the Group Specialty Council of American Psychological Association

Addressing Diversity Dynamics in Group Therapy

This book illustrates group dynamics and group interventions in response to diversity-related content and processes in group therapy.

Perspectives informed by conceptual frameworks guide the discussion of specific clinical interventions and the implications for training. Cultural dimensions of race, international heritage, classism, religion, and aspects of intersectionality associated with these dimensions are a particular emphasis. Key sections for each chapter include Conceptual Framework, Group Interventions, Teaching or Case Examples, Intersectionality, Ethical Considerations, and Implications for Training and/or Practice. Professional development opportunities for mental health professionals as well as training implications for psychiatry residents and psychology interns is addressed, and case studies offer practical examples for guiding therapists and trainees to intervene more effectively in addressing diversity dynamics in group therapy.

An important and timely resource that belongs in every group practitioner's repertoire, this resource is broad enough to be integrated into a course for a training or graduate program and specific enough to serve as a shelf reference for those in practice.

Alexis Abernethy, Ph.D. is a clinical psychologist and professor of psychology in the School of Psychology & Marriage and Family Therapy at Fuller Theological Seminary. In 2021 she was named chief academic officer at Fuller.

AGPA Group Therapy Training and Practice Series
Series Editors: Les Greene and Rebecca MacNair-Semands

The American Group Psychotherapy Association (AGPA) is the foremost professional associ-ation dedicated to the field of group psychotherapy, operating through a tri-partite structure: AGPA, a professional and educational organization; the Group Foundation for Advancing Mental Health, its philanthropic arm; and the International Board for Certification of Group Psychotherapists, a standard setting and certifying body. This multidisciplinary association has approximately 3,000 members, including psychiatrists, psychologists, social workers, nurses, clinical mental health counselors, marriage and family therapists, pastoral counse-lors, occupational therapists and creative arts therapists, many of whom have been recog-nized as specialists through the Certified Group Psychotherapist credential. The association has 26 local and regional societies located across the country. Its members are experi-enced mental health professionals who lead psychotherapy groups and various non-clinical groups. Many are organizational specialists who work with businesses, not-for-profit organi-zations, communities and other "natural" groups to help them improve their functioning.

The goal of the AGPA Group Therapy Training and Practice Series is to produce the high-est quality publications to aid the practitioner and student in updating and improving his/her knowledge, professional competence and skills with current and new developments in methods, practice, theory, and research in the group psychotherapy field. Books in this series are the only curriculum guide and resource for a variety of courses credentialed by the Inter-national Board for Certification of Group Psychotherapists. While this is the series' original and primary purpose, the texts are also useful in a variety of other settings including as a resource for students and clinicians interested in learning more about group psychotherapy, as a text in academic courses, or as part of a training curriculum in a practicum or internship training experience.

Books in this Series:

Group Psychotherapy with Children
Core Principles for Effective Practice
by Tony L. Sheppard and Zachary J. Thieneman

Addressing Diversity Dynamics in Group Therapy
Clinical and Training Applications
Edited by Alexis D. Abernethy

For more information about this series, please visit www.routledge.com/AGPA-Group-Therapy-Training-and-Practice-Series/book-series/AGPA.

Addressing Diversity Dynamics in Group Therapy

Clinical and Training Applications

Edited by Alexis D. Abernethy

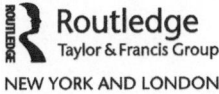
Routledge
Taylor & Francis Group

NEW YORK AND LONDON

Designed cover image: © Getty Images

First published 2025
by Routledge
605 Third Avenue, New York, NY 10158

and by Routledge
4 Park Square, Milton Park, Abingdon, Oxon, OX14 4RN

Routledge is an imprint of the Taylor & Francis Group, an informa business

ISBN: 978-1-032-59687-7 (hbk)
ISBN: 978-1-032-59685-3 (pbk)
ISBN: 978-1-003-45578-3 (ebk)

DOI: 10.4324/9781003455783

Typeset in Optima
by Apex CoVantage, LLC

Contents

Acknowledgments

I deeply appreciate the invitation of the series editors, Drs. MacNair-Semands, Mamarosh, Les Greene, and CEO Angela Stephens to make this contribution. Editing this book provided an opportunity for my reflection on past and more recent diversity training that I have conducted for group therapists. Even more valuable was the opportunity to invite my colleagues to contribute their conceptual, training, and clinical insights. I am deeply indebted to the authors for their thoughtful contributions that have made this work possible. Authors, thank you for your creativity, commitment to improving the field of group therapy, and efforts to serve underrepresented peoples as well as all group members more effectively.

Several chapters refer to training opportunities including institute groups, therapy groups, and experiential training groups that have informed our work. I am so thankful to the participants in these varied groups as the opportunity to lead these groups, to reflect on our leadership, and in some cases obtain feedback from participants has enriched our understanding of and practice of group therapy.

A critical contributor to this work was my project assistant, Anne Wangugi. Anne is a doctoral student in clinical psychology in the School of Psychology & Marriage and Family Therapy at Fuller Theological Seminary. She initially served in a coordinating role in communicating with the authors related to their chapter submission. She also provided copyediting for the submitted chapters. Her work on assuring the references and other style considerations were in APA format, as well as assisting in the final phase of preparing the book for publication was invaluable. My executive assistant, Sukari Waters, also played a significant role in the early and final stages of this project. I am deeply indebted to Anne and Sukari.

Fuller Theological Seminary has been a rich environment for me to teach group therapy and supervise psychology graduate students for 25 years. I have gained important insights from my students over the years that have informed my teaching and training. I am thankful that Dean Emeritus Winston Gooden welcomed me as a new faculty to take a leadership role in group therapy. I have been thankful to have the opportunity to provide consultation to Fuller alumni as they provided experiential process groups for our students for over ten years.

I have been a member of the American Group Psychotherapy Association (AGPA) for over 35 years. I have been formed as a group therapist, process group leader, and organizational leader through AGPA. I am thankful for both the opportunities and challenges that this has presented as it has inspired me to create more space for groups to serve people from all backgrounds in more effective ways. I am thankful to Sherrie Smith, Josephine Cunningham Tervalon, Dr. Eleanor Counselman, Marsha Block, and Angela Stephens for their encouragement over the years.

I was first exposed to group therapy through my clinical psychology internship at Howard University Hospital. Wayman Cunningham was my supervisor and professor. I had the rich opportunity to observe him leading an inpatient and outpatient group weekly. I am so grateful to him as well as Dr. Dorothy Evans Holmes, the Psychology Internship Training Director, who offered an internship with such an in-depth training experience in group therapy.

Finally, I am thankful to my parents, Rev. Rufus S. Abernethy, Jr. and Agnes T. Abernethy as well as my grandmother, Sadye Y. Thomas, who always encouraged my intellectual development and my leadership skills.

With deepest appreciation,
Alexis D. Abernethy

Part 1
Considering Diversity Dynamics

Introduction

Alexis D. Abernethy

Introduction

This book aims to illustrate group dynamics and group interventions in response to diversity-related content and processes in group therapy. Although there are several recent books on diversity in group therapy (Kane et al., 2022; McRae & Short, 2009; Ribeiro, 2020), several of those books have a particular focus such as women and power, social justice, or psychoanalytic theory. A few books (Pelech et al., 2016; Steen et al., 2022) have included a broader focus on multiple social identities or leader interventions with diverse members in the group. This book makes a unique contribution as it offers insights for diversity dimensions that have received less attention—classism, spirituality, and international heritage—and engages these dimensions from a conceptual framework that includes systems-centered approaches and a decolonizing framework. In addition, this contribution emphasizes the implications of these insights for training and providing consultation.

Perspectives that are informed by conceptual frameworks will guide the discussion of specific clinical interventions and the implications for training. Cultural dimensions of race, international heritage, classism, and religion and aspects of intersectionality associated with these dimensions are a particular emphasis. Key sections for each chapter will include the following: *Conceptual Framework, Group Interventions, Teaching or Case Examples, Intersectionality, Ethical Considerations, and Implications for Training and/or Practice*. Professional development opportunities for mental health professionals as well as training implications for psychiatry residents and psychology interns will be addressed. Case examples will offer practical examples for guiding therapists and trainees to intervene more effectively in addressing diversity dynamics in group therapy.

It is hoped that this book will accomplish the following objectives:

1. Contribute to the group psychotherapy literature on addressing diversity in groups.
2. Identify conceptual frameworks that inform culturally competent interventions.
3. Articulate key interventions that increase the responsiveness of group therapists to diversity-related considerations.
4. Illustrate specific challenges and opportunities in exploring similarities and differences in group therapy related to race, religion, class, and international heritage.
5. Consider how intersectionality complicates and clarifies the process of addressing diversity dynamics in group therapy.
6. Clarify training approaches that improve trainees' cultural competence in group therapy.

DOI: 10.4324/9781003455783-2

Overview of the Book

This volume begins with Donna J. Harris, a licensed clinical social worker with over 30 years of clinical practice, contributing a chapter on "Identifying and Working Through Racialized Enactments in Group Psychotherapy." She defines racialized enactments drawing from her clinical experience and also utilizes the literature and her own personal experience to illustrate how these enactments influence the group process. Helpful elements include her articulation of the pervasiveness of racial enactments as well as the tendency to avoid their examination. She identifies the openness of the therapist to nondefensively exploring these enactments as a critical posture in group therapy.

The next contribution, "Undoing Racialized Enactments by Developing a Decolonizing Group Culture and Weakening Closed Survivor Roles" is authored by four scholars: Susan P. Gantt, a psychologist in private practice, Coordinator of group psychotherapy training in psychiatry at Emory University, and Chair of the Systems-Centered Training (SCT) and Research Institute; Willard Ashley, President and CEO of Dr. Willard Ashley, Sr., LLC in Upper Montclair, New Jersey, consultant, coach, trustee, and faculty member of the New Jersey Institute for the Training in Psychoanalysis, and a pastor; Joan Adams, a licensed clinical social worker in Harlem, NY and consultant on race, racism, anti-racism and anti-oppression for organizations, groups and individuals; and Frances Carter, a licensed social worker in the Philadelphia area, a founding member of the Systems-Centered Training and Research Institute, a Board Member and System Mentor with a clinical and consulting practice working with individuals, couples, groups and organizations. These authors build on the concept of racialized enactments and draw from Systems-Centered and anti-racist approaches to address racial dynamics in groups. They argue that all therapists must be attuned to the pervasiveness of racialized dynamics as well as the central role of experiential learning in undoing these enactments. Case examples illustrate both the development of a deepened understanding of the emergence of racism in group dynamics as well as how SCT training groups have enabled racialized dynamics to be explored and in each developmental phase of SCT-informed intervention approaches.

Kristin Miserocchi, a staff psychologist and group coordinator in Mental Health Services at Washington University in St. Louis, MO, and Yujia Lei, a staff psychologist in Habif Health and Wellness Center at the Washington University in St. Louis, contribute the third chapter, "Adopting a Multicultural Orientation to Work with International Students of Color in Heterogeneous Interpersonal Process Groups." These authors use a multicultural orientation (MCO) framework to facilitate the exploration of international students' diverse cultural backgrounds and identities in interpersonal groups. They highlight the heterogeneity and intersectionality of international students and also note frequently shared and common experiences of international students, such as being uprooted from a familiar community and adapting to a new cultural environment. The potential benefit of interpersonal groups for supporting international students is highlighted drawing on the concepts of cultural humility, cultural comfort, and cultural opportunities. The importance of the group therapist facilitating an environment where group members might experience these dimensions is emphasized. Although a MCO framework is recommended for groups including international students, the authors argue that this framework would be a helpful lens for all groups and an effective approach for managing the heterogeneity that is present in all groups.

Cindy Aron, Senior Director of Clinical Services at Ascend Consultation in Healthcare in Chicago, Illinois and an adjunct professor of psychiatry at, University of Wisconsin School of Medicine and Public Health and Sydney Lefay, a consultation-liaison psychiatrist and adjunct assistant professor of psychiatry at Oregon Health & Science University, contribute an important fourth chapter, "Hidden Diversity: The Invisible Oppressor of Classism," that makes visible an often overlooked dimension of diversity. They identify key considerations in classism including the intersection of income, education, and occupation. They emphasize the prevalence of class bias as well as how individuals' perception of their own class may differ from how others perceive them. Although class is an intersectional dimension by itself, it also intersects with other dimensions of culture such as race and gender in varied ways. Group therapists' attentiveness to their own classist biases as well as the tendency for classist dynamics to be ignored or unattended in groups are illustrated through case examples. Intervention approaches are offered that facilitate the examination of these dynamics.

In the fifth chapter, "An Unsacred Silence: Conceptualizing Religious Dynamics in Group Psychotherapy," Mendel Horowitz, a psychotherapist, researcher, and author in Jerusalem who is certified by the International Board for Certification of Group Psychotherapists, and Avidan Milevsky, an associate professor of psychology at Ariel University in Israel and a psychologist at the Center for Mental Health in Israel and at Wellspring Counseling in Towson, Maryland who is a researcher and author, highlight how attentiveness to religious and spiritual backgrounds of group members may enhance group treatment. Drawing on lessons learned from an interpersonal ethnoreligiously heterogenous group in Jerusalem, the authors share principles that are applicable to all groups. They offer a lens that includes the dimensions of ritual, social, and experiential dimensions through which religious dynamics emerge in groups and highlight common transferential and countertransferential resistances to this examination. A rich case example illustrates how the therapist integrated religious values to assist a member in working through his shame and guilt. Varied perspectives offered in the group were also instrumental in facilitating this work.

Experiential Process Groups are essential to group psychotherapy training. Syeda Razia Haider, a fourth-year psychiatry resident at Duke University Hospital, Seamus Bhatt-Mackin, a staff psychiatrist in the Durham Veterans Affairs Health Care System, Director of the Program for Clinical Group Work in the VA Mid-Atlantic Mental Illness Research, Education and Clinic Center, and a Consulting Associate in the Duke University Department of Psychiatry and Behavioral Sciences, and Meenakshi Denduluri, a psychiatrist in private practice in Chicago, discuss "Diversity Considerations in Psychiatry Process Groups: The Medical Doctor as Trainee" focusing on psychiatry residency training. The authors acquaint readers with the context of medical education and particularly the centrality of practicing procedures as a method of learning. The unique features of Psychiatry Training Process Groups are compared to other groups such as T-Groups, Balint Groups, and support groups. Examples where diversity dynamics emerge in process groups illustrate common challenging dynamics as well as helpful approaches for responding to these interactions. The importance of an explicit focus on diversity dynamics in process groups provides a rich training context for residents to be better prepared to manage these issues not only with their peers, but also with their patients.

Haim Weinberg, a licensed psychologist in Israel and California, a group analyst, and Certified Group Psychotherapist in private practice in Sacramento, California offers an opportunity for "Rethinking the Group Leader's Interventions Addressing Diversity" and Winston Gooden, Dean Emeritus of the School of Psychology at Fuller Theological Seminary, and a psychologist in private practice, takes up this offer by responding to his invitation in Chapter seven. Gooden provides an opportunity to see therapists' change in mindset (e.g., openness to incorporating diversity issues in group) as well as resistances (to the full benefit of incorporating a diversity focused lens) to this exploration. He offers a comparison and contrast between traditional group therapy and current approaches that are more attentive to racism and social justice. Weinberg also highlights potential challenges in leading groups that are intended to support marginalized persons. Gooden responds to Weinberg's thesis and provides a different lens for considering the next phase of work in addressing diversity in groups.

Ron Hopson, associate professor of clinical psychology and pastoral care with a joint faculty appointment at Howard University in the Department of Psychology and the School of Divinity and licensed psychologist in Washington casts a conceptual lens for considering diversity approaches in group therapy. His chapter on "The Work of Overcoming Racism/White Supremacy in Group" points out the insidious role of racism that he purposely labels white supremacy. The pervasiveness of this phenomena in our society and groups necessitates a clear reckoning and intentional work and preparation to address white supremacy as a critical element of cultural competence. He draws on the work of Wilfred Bion and Ernest Becker to address racism. He identifies four challenges that, if addressed, offer hope in overcoming racism/white supremacy: 1) denial; 2) impaired empathy; 3) shame; and 4) the fear/denial of death. He uses a case example to illustrate these challenges and shares a sense of hope for the recovery of passion if we can overcome racism/white supremacy.

In the conclusion, I collect these rich resources in a collage of insight and wisdom and discuss more broadly the implications for training. One image is if we ignore these dimensions that have been so richly articulated by these authors. Another image is that we dare to dream a world that makes room for everyone. That we dare to imagine a group that makes more room for everyone. That we embrace the conceptual challenge, the research challenge, the methodological challenge, the intervention challenge and set our course toward a future where group therapy will be a more healing environment for all.

References

Kane, Y. I., Masselink, S. M., & Weiss, A. C. (Eds). (2022). *Women, intersectionality, and power in group psychotherapy leadership.* Routledge/Taylor & Francis Group.

McRae, M. B. & Short, E. L. (2009). *Racial and cultural dynamics in group and organizational life: Crossing boundaries.* Sage Publications, Inc.

Pelech, W., Basso, R., Lee, D. C., & Gandarilla, M. (2016). *Inclusive group work.* Oxford University Press.

Ribeiro, M. D. (Ed.). (2020). *Examining social identities and diversity issues in group therapy: Knocking at the boundaries.* Routledge. https://doi.org/10.4324/9780429022364

Steen, S., Vannatta, R., & Leva, K. (2022). *Introduction to group counseling: A culturally sustaining and inclusive framework.* Springer Publishing.

1 Identifying and Working Through Racialized Enactments in Group Psychotherapy

Donna J. Harris

Conceptual Framework

If the therapy group is a "social microcosm" (Yalom & Leszcz, 2020), the question is not what to do *if* a racialized enactment should occur, but rather how to intervene when one inevitably transpires. It is only recently that mental health professions have begun to acknowledge the need to address not only the intrapsychic phenomena in group and individual therapy, but also the reality of systems of oppression that impact the daily lives of people with marginalized identities. Tummala-Narra (2016) notes that psychoanalytic clinicians have the reputation amongst Black, Indigenous and People of Color (BIPOC) clients of minimizing contextual issues that are critically important to development and mental health. Powell (2018) believes that this "collective silence" limits our ability to explore and treat the effects of race, racism, racialized trauma, and implicit bias, and privilege (p. 1021). It is interesting to note that in the 818 pages of the 6th edition of *The Theory and Practice of Group Psychotherapy* (Yalom & Leszcz, 2020), considered a classic and required reading for anyone interested in group work, there are only two paragraphs on cultural and gender diversity housed under group homogeneity but no mention of working through cultural or racial enactments. How is the neglect of this topic possible in a world that has become increasingly xenophobic and intolerant of racial, ethnic, and religious differences (Bemak & Chung, 2019)?

Some scholars believe that cultural dialogues in group therapy can reduce racial tensions (Bemak & Chung, 2019; Garran et al., 2022; Sue, 2015). Thus, there is a need not to simply become aware of racial tensions in society but to attend to their manifestation as racial enactments in our therapy groups. Leary (2000) uses the term racial enactments to describe interpersonal repetitions in the therapeutic space, that are "interactive sequences that embody the actualization in the clinical situation of cultural attitudes towards race and racial difference" (Leary, p. 640). These enactments have to do with how we have been conditioned and socialized to discuss or more often avoid discussions around race. It is also important to note that these enactments can occur not only in mixed-race but also same race interactions. For example, I was a participant in a two-year program with a mixed-race cohort. One day the facilitator inquired about the silence of one of the participants, an African American woman. She noted that she had given up because even though she had contributed to the conversation, no one seemed to notice, and she felt invisible. When asked what had contributed to this feeling, she explained that she felt it was because she had darker skin. She looked at me and explained that I had lighter-skin privilege and that my proximity to whiteness caused people to engage with me differently than with her. Having never thought of myself as "light skinned" I realized that her observation of the group seemed accurate. All the participants engaged with me on a regular basis and seemed to

DOI: 10.4324/9781003455783-3

value my contributions over hers. Racialized enactments are unconscious processes that mirror social inequities, implicit bias, racism, and internalized racism.

Microaggressions

Another type of racial enactment is a microaggression, a term first coined by Pierce (1978), a black psychiatrist, referring to "subtle, stunning, often automatic, and non-verbal exchanges, which are 'put downs'" (as cited by Friedman, 2019, p. 6). Later, Sue (2007) expanded on the definition, stating that racial microaggressions are "brief and commonplace daily verbal, behavioral, or environmental indignities, whether intentional or unintentional, that communicate hostile, derogatory, or negative racial slights and insults toward people of color" (p. 271). Microaggressions are subtle discriminatory slights that are often outside of the perpetrator's conscious awareness, which, if unaddressed, can have profound negative effects on individuals as well as the group (Miles et al., 2021; Schmidt, 2018).

Sue (2007) identifies three types of microaggressions: microinvalidations, microinsults, and microassaults. Microassaults are the most obvious and can be verbal or nonverbal and are most likely conscious and deliberate. They include racial slurs and avoidant behaviors such as locking a car door when driving in a black neighborhood or waiting on a white customer first even though a person of color arrived before them. Microinsults reflect the dominant traditional white American cultural values, such as individualism and self-reliance (pulling oneself up by one's bootstraps). Microinsults are subtle, often unknown to the perpetrator, can be verbal or nonverbal, and often convey insulting messages to people of color. These include references to people of color being less intelligent or less qualified for a job (Sue et al., 2007). Microinvalidations also tend to be unconscious and covert, and are motivated by stereotypes and implicit bias. These tend to be communications that exclude, deny, or nullify thoughts, feelings, and experiences of people of color. An example would be a client describing discrimination at work and a therapist questioning if there might be other explanations for their experience, suggesting that they may be a bit paranoid.

Until recently, psychodynamic theory implied that attending to social injustices was more in the realm of sociology and that psychologists and analysts should be limited to exploring intrapsychic phenomena (Layton, 2020; Powell, 2018; Tummala-Narra, 2016). Layton with Leavy-Spermous (2020) argue that therapists have actually colluded with a capitalist worldview by artificially separating the individual from their social context. The title of Sue et al.'s article "Microaggressions in Everyday Life" speaks to the insidious nature of these aggressions on people of color. They occur daily, in a variety of settings, by various people, including clinicians. It is likely that therapists conduct their ordinary practice while unintentionally conveying deeply ingrained biases and values to clients of color in various ways that are experienced as racial microaggressions. There are many resources available for group therapists (Singh et al., 2012) to consider the societal context as critical dimensions not only in the lives of group members, but also in the group process (Miles et al., 2021).

In the United States, it seems inevitable that racial enactments are destined to occur in diverse groups in social, educational, and professional settings. Conversations about race and marginalized identities are inherently challenging due to our society's extensive history around race, power, and exclusion. Unfortunately, this often results in outright avoidance or painful "tippy toeing" around what are considered delicate subjects for fear of offending or "othering" group members. Recently, having just returned from a vacation in Mexico, the leader of a group in which I am a participant carefully inquired whether it was appropriate to comment on the tan I had acquired. The group anxiously awaited my response, which was to burst out laughing and to say "yes, black people tan." If only everyone risked inquiring about the appropriateness of a comment! If this had occurred with a stranger, I might not have responded with a sense of humor. This example stresses the importance of establishing a trusting relationship. It was also important that the facilitator asked if it was an appropriate comment, suggesting his awareness of potential microaggressions.

Like Leary (2000), I propose that racial enactments offer the opportunity to open important clinical discoveries because, if not effectively addressed, they can derail the process completely. In the example above the facilitator was open and transparent about the potential of his comment being inappropriate. There was room and an invitation for me to say "no" and to express whatever feelings emerged for me. Leary (2000) suggests that perhaps the most common racial enactment has been our silence about racial issues.

Racial Dynamics

There are many potential barriers to effective engagement around race, microaggressions, and cross-cultural dialogue. First, because these enactments involve implicit biases, they may largely operate out of clinicians' awareness. Garran et al. (2022) identify three major obstacles in clinical work: racial dynamics, internalized racism, and inattention to issues of power and privilege.

Given a larger sociocultural context of racism, racial dynamics include a common concern related to not wanting to be labeled racist and consequently avoiding the topic altogether. Most clinicians do not want to be "the oppressor" or associated with racist, sexist or heterosexist beliefs. Despite helfpul resources on white privilege, systemic racism, and oppression, therapists remain fearful of addressing these issues in their groups. Identifying biases and microaggressions is also challenging in that they are closely aligned with our social identities as well as our strong emotions related to power, privilege, and oppression (Miles et al., 2021). The issue of seemingly not noticing color is not exclusive to white practitioners. Therapists of color may also fail to explore the meaning of a client's race or ethnicity, or the impact of race on their lives, which can be due to internalized racism and white supremacy or their own painful experiences.

On the opposite side of the spectrum are clinicians who overemphasize the importance of race and ethnicity, or who awkwardly raise the topic, insisting that the client needs to explore how race impacts them inside and outside of the therapeutic space. Some clinicians may overemphasize socio-political problems by focusing solely on race while missing the complex intersection between social identities and oppressive systems.

Internalized Racism

This term can refer to either internalized feelings of racial superiority, or feelings of being "less than" based on one's race, or even taking responsibility for one's own social oppression (Garran et al., 2022). One might suspect internalized racism when a BIPOC seeks out a white therapist because they believe they have superior training and skill to a BIPOC clinician. White clinicians often profess that they have few clients of color and attribute this to BIPOCs not believing in therapy, rather than being accountable for the part they may play. A white male therapist may take on a position of authority and expertise in making interpretations in the group, ignoring what women or people of color are trying to convey, thus invalidating their contributions. In addition, internalized racism can appear as hatred or distancing from one's own race.

Power Dynamics

In addition to societal and political issues, there is an inherent power differential between therapist and client. Although this power dynamic may be more complicated when a white male patient or native English speaking patient is being seen by a female Latina bilingual therapist, this power differential remains a consideration. Clinicians must be attuned to the power and privilege they experience associated with race, education, income, etc. Therapists may unwittingly reenact societal power dynamics in the larger society. For instance, a female therapist may allow a white male to dominate the group, or a clinician of color may make assumptions of sameness about a group member of the same racial group, causing them to miss important power differences.

Group Interventions

Therapeutic Posture

Prior to addressing specific interventions with cultural enactments, it is of equal importance to note that, first and foremost, group practitioners need to invite discussion around racialized and other marginalized identities. If a group therapist is not inclined to think of themselves in racialized terms, they may omit welcoming this discussion from participants. The easiest way to do this is to allude to one's own racial identity, as a form of disclosure. For example, "As a black woman, my experience is . . ." This simple task is often neglected by white therapists who aren't used to thinking of themselves in racialized terms but can also be avoided by people of color not wanting to draw attention to their own racial identity as being different from the group.

Microaggressions need to be recognized before deciding how to respond. Here, a mindful approach is useful, which involves tuning into one's own emotional and physical reactions, then observing the room and trying to ascertain the impact on others by taking a closer look at members' facial and bodily expressions. A response is necessary, even if a group member has already reacted. It is the group leader's responsibility as the person with the most power in the room to name the microaggression and respond in some way. This step is essential in developing trust and modeling appropriate responses to cultural enactments. As the group becomes more cohesive and experienced, there will be a mutual responsibility in such responses as members learn how to address microaggressions following the leader's example. The therapist's response involves self-reflection, observation, and both therapeutic and ethical decision-making (Lefforge et al., 2020). There is mutuality in this process, as the therapist also needs to take into consideration the response as a group and as individuals.

Another dilemma the therapist faces is who to respond to first in a cross-cultural exchange where there has been an enactment that has caused strong feelings. Therapists must consider the socio-political context in which the interaction is taking place and the identities and privileges of the participants. Attending to feelings of marginalization or othering is of the utmost importance. Thus, it is good practice to first check in with the person who was "microaggressed" upon before moving to curiosity about what was expressed. Most often, this is a person with a marginalized identity. Therapists who fail to attend to the person experiencing the microaggression risk repeating and perpetuating harmful cultural enactments. It should be noted that sometimes this just happens, as we are all humans who at times, lack awareness. If a group member should expose the therapist's failure to intervene, it is vital to absorb the feedback and resist a defensive response.

What is extremely helpful to the group is for the therapist to admit their mistake. This, too, is important modeling for group members who will inevitably become involved in misunderstandings.

How one responds to a microaggression depends on the participants and their associated power dynamics. For instance, a group member of color once accused me, a black group therapist, of "acting white". The accusation of performing whiteness may be one of the most hurtful things an African American can say to another. It is a slight which is often hurled at educated people of color who, by virtue of their education, how they speak or present themselves, may be perceived as "sell-outs" to the Black community. This enactment involved multiple layers of complexity, not only of racial and power dynamics but also transference reactions from the client who clearly experienced me as prioritizing a white person over them. As a relational therapist, I also had to question whether there was some truth in this person's experience. As an African American woman, I have become quite adept at making white people feel comfortable and this tendency might have played out in group, making the person of color feel invisible or overlooked.

In this case, it was important for me to verbalize that possibility and to invite the group members to look at the interaction together. Only through this mutual process were we able to determine that the person of color and the white person had spoken at the same time and many of the group members had only heard one of them, the white person. The group did acknowledge however that this selective attention in and of itself might very well have been enactment of privileging a white person over a person of color.

Responding to a racial enactment requires the practitioner to do something which may be counterintuitive, based on most theoretical models. They must allow the socio-cultural reality to take precedence over intrapsychic processes. They must name the microaggression and define it within the context of power dynamics common in interracial encounters, whereby a member of the dominant group degrades or applies a stereotype to a member of a marginalized group (Schmidt, 2018). As stated earlier, silence is not an option here, and people of color should not be put in the position to explain what occurred. In mature groups, another member might name the enactment, but in earlier stages of group development this is not usually the case.

After the therapist identifies the enactment, feelings can then be solicited from group members. If it is a white person who has committed the slight, Schmidt (2018) suggests that the group leader assists them in understanding the impact of racial slights on people of color. If the individual finds it hard to understand or accept that harm was perpetrated, then the leader can use a broader frame around systemic oppression to illustrate how individuals are influenced by broader society. The leader's acknowledgment of a microaggression models an appropriate response to the group and validates the experience of the person who has been impacted. The goal eventually is for group members to become more cognizant of these interpersonal slights and to be able to address them as they manifest in group sessions. In addition to naming microaggressions, the leader must attend to the impact on individuals as well as on the group while acknowledging the socio-cultural-political context.

In addition to microaggressions, the process group has proven fertile ground for other types of cultural enactments. For example, when a group member is singled out because of curiosity about their background, religion, or other aspect of their identity, initially this interaction seems positive. Group members are getting to know one another, posing questions, and somehow suggesting that they are exceptional in some way. This can feel flattering to the member in the role of the "other," and they may even respond with gratitude that people are interested in their unique experience. On the other hand, many of my BIPOC clients have reported feeling used as the interest does not feel genuine or authentic. As a black woman who often functions in predominately white spaces, this often happens to me, but it ends up highlighting the problem (a lack of diverse voices) when white people are so eager to hear from me, one of the few BIPOC in these spaces.

Cultural transference and countertransference dynamics also play a part in contributing to challenges related to cultural differences. Reliance on a purely clinical theory can be used to defend against the exploration and identification of sociocultural tensions (Garran et al., 2022). When this happens, the message to clients is that the exploration of racial enactments is outside the realm of therapy and should be done elsewhere.

Although this chapter mostly refers to racialized enactments, there is the potential for many types of cultural enactments to occur in therapeutic and support groups. Garran et al. (2022) discuss the notion of agent vs target social identities, with the former being more privileged than the latter[1]. This complex matrix of agent-target identities is alive and well in the group social microcosm, as participants are often aware of both. For instance, while I identify as an African American woman, there are also Europeans and Ashkenazi Jews in my ancestry. Thus, I come from a history of enslavement, antisemitism, and perpetrators of oppressive acts from the European side. This intergenerational trauma of both oppressed and oppressor resides in the DNA of many people of color (DeGruy, 2005; Gump, 2017).

Intervention Models

Group therapy draws from several theoretical traditions, all of which have been largely influenced by the experiences of white European and European American researchers and practitioners. Those of us who lead multicultural and BIPOC groups incorporate techniques from many sources in order to effectively address cultural enactments and provide affirming therapeutic interventions to people with marginalized identities. My work is informed first and foremost by my training in Clinical Social Work and Relational Psychoanalysis, where I learned to be client centered and embrace the notion of mutuality in the treatment room, thus allowing me to relinquish the notion of being the expert in the room and instead embracing the influence of my clients. In addition, I've been greatly influenced by Critical Race Theory (CRT), a post-modern, client-centered framework that attends to both systemic and individual oppression. CRT encourages me to observe the intersection of multiple identities in groups and encourages transformation through dialogue and social relationships (Ortiz & Jani, 2010). Principles of mindfulness have been instrumental in encouraging me to take my time and be more attuned to the mind and body in the here and now.

There are several models of practice that offer effective ways to encourage open discussions about race and address cultural enactments. Sue (2015) proposes a set of eleven actions when conducting "race talk". These include understanding one's own identity and self as a racial/cultural being; openness to having and admitting racial biases; becoming comfortable discussing race and racism; being able to deconstruct symbolic meaning of emotions; the ability to validate and facilitate discussion around feelings related to oppression and race; discerning the process versus the content of race talk; commenting on process in difficult dialogues; not allowing group members to stew in silence when a challenging dialogue occurs; understanding that communication can be culture bound; preparing participants for difficult dialogues; and, feeling discomfort and validating and encouraging members when they engage in difficult dialogue.

The suggestions mentioned above are all excellent, but they are not enough. Clinicians require ongoing practice to develop a degree of comfort in addressing racialized enactments. Part of this requires them to intentionally create multicultural groups! Often, groups consist of several white members and one lone person of color if any at all. Furthermore, engaging in cross-cultural dialogues in mixed groups is challenging and requires specialized training and ongoing experience. The approach that I have found most useful in helping group members engage with each other around race and other experiences of marginalization is "Mindful Facilitation", a skill set created by filmmaker/therapist Lee Mun Wah (2011). It is a trauma-informed, culturally responsive model which encourages people to have challenging conversations with one another around differences in race, ethnicity, and other social identities. After becoming certified in this technique, I modified it specifically for clinicians practicing individual and group therapy. As with all the strategies mentioned in this chapter, Mindful Facilitation begins with the clinician becoming aware of their own biases. They are encouraged to be "mindful" of their emotions, bodily sensations, and the impact of the client's words on them, from the point of view of their own social identity. Thus, as a black woman, I am aware of a tightening in my chest when a person says "I don't mean to offend, but. . .". The reason for this is usually because when a person makes such a statement, they proceed to offend someone. An illustration of Mindful Facilitation will be given in Case one below.

Case Examples

Case 1: Is that a Microaggression?

In an online workshop on engaging in groups, I showed a video clip from the film *The Color of Fear* (1994) directed by Lee Mun Wah. This documentary depicts eight men engaged in conversations about race and identity, and takes place in Ukiah, California, over the course of a weekend. There are two Asian Americans, two European Americans, two Latinos, and two African American men. In this clip, Victor, an African American man, becomes angry with a white participant, David, who had suggested that perhaps Victor and "his people" were going the "wrong way" and not taking advantage of opportunities available to them. It is a very emotionally intense and impactful clip. After the viewing, the following dialogue occurred:

> Donna to the group: "So, what came up for you in watching this clip? How did it impact you?"
> Jennifer, an older white woman: "Wow! Victor was just so articulate!"
> (The participants have non-verbal reactions, looking away, frozen, silent.)
> Stephanie, another white participant, types in the chat: "Donna is that a microaggression?"

My feelings were multilayered, and I froze for what seemed like an eternity. In terms of countertransference, I recognized my anger—not at the question, because it seemed appropriate given the situation, but because of how it was posed in secret. I realized that had we been in-person, this could not have transpired in this manner, and wondered if this participant would have said anything at all.

Another way of thinking about microaggressions is as a form of enactment. In the preceding vignette, the description of a black man as "articulate" is fraught with stereotypical references to the inferiority of African Americans, who were thought to be less intelligent than whites. Then, there was a bystander response which was delivered in an indirect, clandestine manner (via text chat), with an implied plea to the facilitator of "you deal with this." As an African American woman who happened to be the group leader, it fell on me to expose the potentially harmful microaggression, thus assuming all the related emotional labor. I refused to take on my assigned role of whistle-blower and instead requested that the bystander verbally articulate her query.

How to intervene? I could wait and see if any of the group members would address the issue. Everyone was frozen, including the one person of color in the group. I could have asked the group, "What just happened?" which is a Mindful Facilitation group intervention, a technique I was in the process of teaching them. I feared that no one would respond. I was experiencing a lot of feelings of my own and was concerned that I would sound angry or accusatory. To respond to the chat would not only be collusion, but it would also avoid the issue. What had transpired was a microaggression, more specifically, a microinsult which Sue et al. (2007) defined as a "subtle snub, frequently unknown to the perpetrator, but clearly conveying a hidden insulting message to the recipient of color" (p. 274).

The least desirable choice would have been to do nothing and to continue with my agenda. Avoidance can in and of itself be considered a form of microaggression. Neville et al. (2013), in their discussion on avoiding discussions of power differences, suggest that this invalidates the lived experiences of Black, Brown, and Indigenous people of color (BIPOC). In this case, other than myself, there was only one BIPOC present, which can be an isolating experience. With diverse groups, it is necessary to process the slight. Not doing so could lead to a cultural rupture without the benefit of reparative experience. For this group, it was a teachable moment, one in which they could observe how to navigate a discussion about microaggression, one of the objectives of the workshop. I decided to address the issue directly:

Donna: "Stephanie, I wonder if you would verbalize the question you put in the chat?"

(Pause, awkward silence, and the group members all look to Stephanie, who begins to speak with hesitation, carefully choosing her words.)

Stephanie: "I could be wrong, Jennifer, but I wonder if what you said could possibly be considered a microaggression?"

Jennifer, looking horrified: "Yes, I knew it as soon as it came out of my mouth! I can't believe I said that!"

With the microaggression having been identified, the group could proceed. Prior to intervening, I took a moment to observe what I was feeling. My chest was tight, and I purposefully relaxed my shoulders by taking a couple of deep breaths. Too often, therapists feel pressured to respond immediately but taking time to attune to oneself as well as others is a vital first step (Bemak & Chung, 2019; Lee, 2011; Sue, 2015). When tracking group members, I am assessing their non-verbal reactions. Do they seem surprised, shocked, angry or are there allies in the room? Also, if there is only one BIPOC participant, which was the case here, I am careful not to call on them first. It is vital for white members to become aware of racial slights and microaggressions as this experience is extremely validating for people with marginalized identities in the room. I then went around the room and asked what came up for people as they witnessed this interaction which turned out to be an excellent opportunity to actively demonstrate the Mindful Facilitation skills we had just reviewed. The group process was very impactful during the last 30 minutes of the workshop. And for the one person of color, it was very important because they had never experienced a white person intervening on their behalf. In this case, the group took on the role of bystander, and one member chose to secretly (via chat) question the slight. These 30 minutes proved invaluable for the entire group. This vignette highlights the importance of the therapist being attuned to the potential emergence of microaggressions.

Case 2: Nice White Man

DiAngelo (2021) describes the subtle forms of "nice racism" perpetrated by self-righteous, "progressive whites" who see themselves as racially sensitive with good intentions. As with microaggressions, nice racism is difficult to prove or challenge. This is because people often equate racism with overt acts designed to cause harm or someone who openly espouses white supremacy. Di Angelo states "the degree to which we see ourselves as not racist, we are going to be very defensive about any suggestion to the contrary" (p. 6) "We see ourselves as outside of the problem." (p. 7). Among the many examples of problematic behaviors described by DiAngelo is the tendency to demonstrate "niceness" by describing one's proximity to people of color or knowledge of black art, sports, etc.

An example of this occurred in a therapy group in which a white male was introducing himself to a diverse group of several women of color, several white men, and several white women. Everyone had taken turns sharing their name and what they hoped to get out of the group. A couple of people commented on how pleased they were that the group was so diverse. Eric had already introduced himself and stated where he was currently living, but then interrupted one of the women of color.

Eric, appearing anxious, says, "I want to share something else about myself, and I'm not sure if it's ok, or not but I really want to take that risk, but I don't want to offend anyone, but I wanted to share that I really like basketball! But you know I didn't want anyone to take offense about me saying that."

The group stared at him in silence, I tried to read the room, paying close attention to the people of color. Some members rolled their eyes . . .

Eric continued, breaking the silence: "I know it might not have been the right thing to say, and I'm not racist or anything; it's just that I like basketball and wanted you all to know something about me, to share—isn't that why we're here?"

Yolanda, a woman of color, interrupted, saying: "Okay! We get it, you like basketball! Don't know why that was important, but whatever!"

Stacey, a white woman, responded, joining Yolanda, "It just seems a bit weird—you are volunteering that, especially when you thought it might be offensive."

Rhonda, a black woman, came to Eric's defense, saying, "I think he was just trying to say something personal for people to get to know him."

From the look on his face and the hesitancy with which he raised the topic of liking to play basketball, it was clear that Eric thought this might be problematic, even offensive to the people of color in the room and in a way, he was attempting to connect with them through the stereotypical notion that all black people like basketball! In fact, Eric went on to describe himself as having taken a risk because of his desire to connect with the group! He then quickly fell into the role of misunderstood victim because he was disappointed that people didn't just see him as a "nice guy."

The cultural enactment here unfolded in many ways. A white male tried to connect with the group by sharing an interest that he assumed might be offensive to the BIPOC members, knowing that it can be a stereotype (all black people like basketball). Yolanda, a BIPOC participant, seemed offended, but didn't specify how she was feeling. Instead, she dismissed him, saying, "whatever." Stacy, a white woman, allied with Yolanda saying, "it was weird," but didn't name the issue (racism), and finally, Rhonda, a black woman, swooped in to protect Eric from his fragility, offering an alternative explanation to the group: "he's just trying to say something personal". Thus, in the first 15 minutes of a new group, there was a stereotype associated with black people expressed, offense taken indirectly by dismissing the person and finally a BIPOC person displaying the need to protect a white male, which could be an expression of internalized white supremacy.

This denial of racism also serves to shield the group from feelings of discomfort that often arise when engaging in dialogues about race. According to DiAngelo (2021) "characteristics of a culture of niceness include white solidarity, avoiding causing or experiencing social discomfort, focusing on connections and commonalities, privileging the concern for perpetrators of racism over the victims, helping others to maintain face, and elevating intentions over impact" (p. 49). Unfortunately, these are strategies which have also been internalized by BIPOC in order to avoid racial tension and conflict.

Given that this was our first session, it is understandable that the group participants avoided "calling out" Eric. They were still getting to know each other and me. As the facilitator, I felt it wise to gently address the issue by slowing down the process and inquiring about Eric's feelings. At first, he denied having any feelings, then he admitted he was anxious and wanted people to like him. It seemed especially important for him to be liked by the women of color in the group. This dynamic of European Americans wanting the approval of people of color is quite familiar and serves as a validation of sorts—a confirmation that a white person is good (i.e., not racist). It serves to benefit the person from the dominant group, but for BIPOCs, this need for assurance can be exhausting.

I noticed one of the women of color looking away and asked her how Eric's initial comment about basketball had impacted her. She initially shrugged it off saying she didn't really feel any way at all, but then said she was annoyed that he assumed that they would be interested in basketball! I asked the group if they were aware of the stereotype of black people playing and being interested in basketball. The group continued to discuss how to handle these microaggressions when they occur. Eric did initially withdraw, feeling shame, but eventually was able to participate in the ensuing conversation. Processing this type of exchange early in the group is challenging, but critical to understanding the group process and modeling how to address microaggressions.

Case 3: Nobody will ever "get me"

This case serves to differentiate when and how the therapist sees what is going on as 'othering' as opposed to cultural exploration. This small process group which included several men, a few men of color and a white man, and several women, including a few women of color and a white woman, was led by a black woman facilitator. Early in the group's development, people engaged in conversations around identity, race, class, and religion as well as agent and target identities. For example, a black woman whose agent status is privileged by her profession as a physician, a white woman who grew up poor, and so on.

One of the members, Efrayim, was visibly different from other group members in terms of his overall presentation. He was dressed as an Orthodox Jew. Efrayim said that no one could truly understand him as an Ultra-Orthodox Jew, but he indicated that he was happy to have the opportunity of a lifetime, to be in such a diverse group, and that he would not be able to do this if we weren't meeting virtually. He also invited the group to ask any questions they might have, given that he was sure he was an enigma. In that session, most members joined in the conversation about feeling different in some way.

As the facilitator, I became aware of a countertransferential urge to engage in what is commonly referred to as "credentialing." I stifled an urge to blurt out that I had worked at Wurzweiler School of Social Work, housed in Yeshiva University in New York, as proof that I was very knowledgeable about Orthodox Jewish practices! Fortunately, a group member was talking, saving me from this common blunder.

During our next session, the group became fascinated with Efrayim, asking questions about Judaism, his family traditions, and his community. Most members admitted having very little knowledge about Judaism, let alone Orthodox practices. Efrayim became the center of attention and I soon became aware that it felt like I was watching a spectacle. What seemed at first to be simple curiosity that he himself had invited the week prior, now seemed voyeuristic, almost like a fetishism. Efrayim's predicament of "nobody will ever get me" was playing out in our group dynamics.

I asked the group what they felt was happening. They looked at me, perplexed, and I shared my discomfort and asked Efrayim how he felt. He shrugged but then shared that it was beginning to feel uncomfortable but that he didn't see a way out since he had invited people's curiosity. I noted how it seemed like people were overly fixated on him and that perhaps they were in some way "othering" Efrayim. In this case, while Efrayim possessed the agent identities of a white male, his religion was a more targeted or marginalized identity. This more highly visible and marginalized identity connected him with other religious minorities such as Muslim women wearing a veil or hijab, Sikh men who adorn turban, or bindis (the decorative mark worn on the forehead of some Hindu women). Any religious attire that differs from the dominant culture is open to curiosity, at best or fear, avoidance, discrimination, and attack at worst. This dynamic is reminiscent of what DiAngelo (2021) refers to as "color-celebrate" credentialling that amplifies racial difference, only in this case it was a hyper focusing on a group member's religion (p. 64). It is for this reason that so many people with marginalized identities are reluctant to join organizational committees created to focus on inclusivity. Most don't want to have to "represent" the LGBTQ or racial perspective because it quickly leads to generalization and stereotyping.

Applying the model of Mindful Facilitation, the first step is self-awareness, I did a quick body scan, making note of the tension in my chest, then I looked around the room, or in this case the online squares, observing non-verbal cues as well as tone. The next step in this process involves affirming what is most important to the person speaking. In other words, observing their words, affect and body language for signs of strong affect. Once the clinician has noted one or two things especially important to the client, they then provide a reflection. An effective reflection captures something meaningful that a person has said, using their own words and positionality. For instance, a good reflection to Efrayim would be, "Efrayim, what I heard you say is that as an Orthodox Jewish man, you don't feel like anyone gets you."

Thus, a clinician may combine a reflection with an expression of empathy and then continue with an inquiry. With the example above, the clinician has already expressed a reflection. Let's assume that the group members continued asking him questions. An inquiry might be:

"Efrayim, what came up for you as a Jewish man when everyone began questioning your religious practices?"

Note that the question specifically incorporates an aspect of the person's identity, in this case, religion, in addressing the religious enactment taking place in this group. There are several individual inquiries designed to deepen a person's affect, and specific group inquiries to help group members become more culturally sensitive and responsive to each other. They include questions about anger, hurt, whether the situation is familiar to the person, and the impact of the situation in the past and in the here and now.

Intersectionality

One of the important insights related to intersectionality is the notion that diversity, equity, and inclusion are more than simply recruiting more people of color into our traditional process group structure. The concept of intersectionality (Crenshaw, 1989) addresses how overlapping systems of oppression faced by individuals with marginalized identities (such as race, gender, religion, ability, and sexual orientation) make it challenging to discern what aspect of their identity is being targeted and how to respond. The dynamics of power, privilege, and oppression need to be addressed. Openness to multiple understandings and perspectives is critical.

For instance, racially, I am an African American, cis-gender, female-identified person, who immigrated to Belgium, where I acculturated and became fluent in French and the customs of the land, while my recently separated mother struggled to put food on the table. I am also bi-sexual but have been in a monogamous heterosexual marriage with a white man for 35 years. How can I possibly separate and silo my experiences related to the various aspects of my identity? No doubt they are all playing out at once at any given time. In my life alone, there is a complex matrix of visible and invisible identities, some with privilege, others that are marginalized, and these aspects have evolved and changed over time. In the United States, I've experienced, on one hand, the privilege of higher education, and on the other anti-black racism and discrimination. In Europe, I was privileged as a U.S. citizen, but experienced colonialistic slurs when mistaken for someone from the then Belgian Congo.

Nayak (2021) reminds us that intersectionality was born out of Crenshaw's (1989) examination of cases involving groups of black women facing discrimination in the workplace as a framework. Intersectionality emerged from the multiple oppressions encountered by black women who simultaneously faced racism and sexism at the 'intersection' of both phenomena. Contrary to popular belief, intersectionality is not about multiple social identities or what is commonly known as the "oppression olympics," whereby people compete over who is the most marginalized. In recent years, the concept has been broadened and includes other oppressive structures, such as ageism, transphobia, homophobia, and discrimination associated with disability (Stevenson, 2020).

Lefforge et al. (2020) discusses that the way one perceives and responds to microaggressions is largely dependent on the intersection of our various social identities, as well as which identity is most salient in the moment. A brown lesbian Latina in a predominately white college may be most aware of her racial identification, as there are likely other members of the LGBTQ community on campus. Alternatively, an encounter with a white male professor may activate feelings about gender.

The concept of intersectional microaggressions (Lefforge et al., 2020) might include stereotypes related to race and class (associating black men with criminality), conflating gender and sexual orientation (assuming all transgender people are gay), perceiving Asian Americans as being good in science and math but otherwise invisible, or objectifying Asian and Middle Eastern women by perceiving them as exotic, subservient, and alluring.

Stevenson (2020) stresses the importance for all clinicians to understand their positionality and social privilege and to consider how that impacts those we invite into or exclude from our psychotherapy groups. Clinicians must "engage with social barriers associated with marginalization that drive the othering that so very dangerously harms people from these marginalized groups when such dynamics inevitably emerge in the matrix" (p. 15).

Ethical Considerations

All mental health professions abide by ethical codes, most of which stipulate the need to work with people from various cultural backgrounds. The National Association of Social

Workers developed a set of Standards and Indicators of Cultural Competency, originally published in 2001. These standards include self-awareness, cross-cultural knowledge and skills, knowledge of services for diverse populations, advocating for diversity in the workplace, education, and training, advocating services to be provided in the language spoken by clients, and promoting diversity in leadership. These are all concepts with which most of us agree, but the notion of cultural competency suggests an endpoint at which one achieves proficiency in serving diverse populations rather than highlighting a lifelong process. It also does not address the inadequacy of our psychological theories which do not account for socio-cultural experiences and the impact of historical and intergenerational trauma.

In recent years, scholars and practitioners have found it more helpful to think in terms of working to become culturally responsive (Lefforge et al., 2020; Miles et al., 2021). Even though group therapists, researchers, and theorists have begun to acknowledge systems of power and oppression, and the need to become more proficient in engaging in dialogues about racial and other identity differences, there remains a dearth of literature in this area (Miles et al., 2021). This limitation, to effectively engage groups in discussions around race and oppression, is not limited to white practitioners. Contrary to popular belief, Black, Brown, and Indigenous People of Color (BBIPOC) and Asian Pacific Islander Desi American clinicians may also avoid taking a deeper dive into the foray of cross-cultural dialogue. This reluctance is often different than with white clinicians and may be due to internalized racism or prior unsuccessful attempts to call attention to racism.

Regardless of cultural background, culturally responsive group therapists have an ethical obligation to address racialized enactments in therapy. However, group therapists are often reluctant to step into a conversation that may go awry and become emotionally volatile. Many fear exposing or confronting racist and bigoted views of group members and causing a rupture in the group. Lastly, there is a very strong concern related to doing harm. Gitterman (2019) asserts that if group leaders aren't proactive in addressing systems of oppression in treatment, it could replicate the trauma of marginalized experience and decrease the possibility for repair and working through it. Bemak and Chung (2019) believe that successfully navigating ethnic and cultural dialogues in a group is essential and can play a significant role, not only in terms of group cohesiveness, but in mitigating racial tensions in general. One of the challenges is that diverse groups have members who are both recipients and perpetrators of racism, oppression, and marginalization, leading to a significant impact on group dynamics.

Implications for Training and Practice

In order to be an ethical and effective group therapist, clinicians need to first develop awareness of systemic issues of racism and oppression in our society, as well as knowledge of the centuries of genocide, subjugation, enslavement and oppression experienced by BIPOC people in North America. It is a mistake to deny the psychological impact that historical and racial trauma has had on all people in this country. The legacy of slavery and oppression continues in our laws, policies, and practices, including in our clinical theories of practice. Thus, clinicians must learn to question the supposed universality of evidence-based theories and research conducted primarily on white college students. Our practice theories and interventions are not inclusive if they have not considered people from diverse backgrounds in terms of race, age, ability, sexual orientation, and immigration status, to name a few.

This awareness and knowledge provides the necessary context to have empathy around experiences of identity-based discrimination and marginalization, which some therapists may not have experienced themselves. Examining issues of power, privilege, and oppression can be personally challenging and uncomfortable. Developing these skills and competencies needs to be ongoing, as opposed to being limited to one diversity or antiracism workshop.

In addition to developing awareness of systemic issues, next steps include exploring personal implicit and explicit biases. This can be done independently using workbooks such as Debbie Irving's excellent book "Waking up White" (2014). However, this exploration is most effective within interpersonal contexts. In other words, to understand diversity one must have sustained interactions with people from different backgrounds. This requires in-depth conversations about different social identities and experiences, something which is usually avoided. Some barriers to intercultural conversations include fear of getting it wrong, or of being offensive, not wanting to be perceived as a racist, feelings of shame and guilt, past experiences of misunderstandings, or being a silent bystander. Given internet accessibility, many racial dialoguing experiences are available via online training, group discussions, book clubs, and workshops—all in the comfort of one's own home.

Adapting a developmental perspective in our understanding of racial identity is essential. As Beverly Tatum (2017) reminds us, the way we conceive of identity and race is an ever-evolving process that continues throughout the lifespan. People living in homogenous neighborhoods who have very limited experiences with diverse people will naturally have less experience understanding the complex dynamics in cross-cultural encounters. Tatum stresses that everyone goes through some type of developmental process with different stages and tasks depending on one's racial background. Her latest edition also acknowledges multiracial families and their unique identity development. As a group facilitator and trainer, it is essential for me to keep racial identity formation theories in mind when I become impatient with people who have less exposure to different cultures. It is equally important to remind myself that although someone may share my racial identity, it does not mean that I understand their experience in the world; resisting assumptions and generalizations is essential.

Derald Wing Sue (2007, 2015) proposed several objectives for working with racial microaggressions, including the need for therapists to do their own work, such as seeking out new experiences with diverse people and validating feelings related to social identity. Miles et al. (2021) suggest additional strategies tailored specifically to group therapeutic encounters, including adapting a multicultural orientation from the pre-group encounter to establish discussions around difference as a norm. Other recommendations are the enhancement of clinical training to include multicultural group facilitation skills and the application of bystander intervention research.

Christine Schmidt (2018), who regularly co-facilitates racial literacy groups as well as groups on whiteness, agrees that there needs to be more training groups for therapists to acquire multicultural intervention skills. She advocates co-facilitation of mixed-race groups with leaders of different racial identities. This approach takes advantage of the therapist's different identities in an effort to minimize implicit biases in each other's interventions.

Conclusion

Although challenging, it can be a very satisfying task for the group therapist to help clients recognize and work through cultural enactments. It requires us to be forever vigilant in systemically examining our unconscious biases, privilege, and complicity with systems of oppression. As a profession, "we recognize the limitations of earlier models and expand our thinking to include spiritual, multiculturalist, and social justice dimensions (Yalom & Leszcz, 2020, p. 133). Our goal should be to do more than give lip service to aspirations of social justice but rather to acknowledge that we haven't done enough to be truly inclusive in our practices. It's certainly worth the risk.

Endnote

1 Agent identities have social statuses that are more privileged by society and reflect dominant values and norms. These privileged identities tend to be unearned. Target identities correspond to social statuses that are more marginalized, where people experience discrimination, exclusion, and oppression. (Garran et al., 2022).

References

Bemak, F, & Chung, C. Y. (2019). Race dialogues in group psychotherapy: Key Issues in training and practice, *International Journal of Group Psychotherapy 69*(2), 172–191. https://doi.org/10.1080/00 207284.2018.1498743.

Crenshaw, K. (1989). Demarginalizing the intersection of race and sex: A Black feminist critique of antidiscrimination doctrine, feminist theory, and antiracist politics. *University of Chicago Legal Forum, 1*(8), 139–167. https://chicagounbound.uchicago.edu/uclf/vol1989/iss1/8

DeGruy, J. (2005). *Post traumatic slave syndrome: America's legacy of enduring injury and healing.* Uptone Press.

DiAngelo, R. (2021). *Nice Racism: How progressive white people perpetuate racial harm.* Beacon Press.

Friedman, S. (2019). Exploration of racial enactments in an interracial therapeutic dyad to foster the strengthening of voice and identity in African American male adolescents. *Smith College Studies in Social Work, 89*(1), 1–17. https://doi.org/10.1080/00377317.2019.1601915

Garran, A. M., Werkmeister Rozas, L., Kang, H., & Miller, J. (2022). *Racism in the United States. Implications for helping professions*, 3rd Edition. Springer Publishing Company, LLC.

Gitterman, P. (2019). Social identities, power, and privilege: The importance of difference in establishing early group cohesion, *International Journal of Group Psychotherapy, 69*(1), 99–125. https://doi.org/10.1080/00207284.2018.1484665.

Gump, J. (2017). The presence of the past: Transmission of slavery's traumas. In: A. Harris, M. Kalb, & S. Klebanoff (Eds), *Demons in the consulting room: Echoes of genocide, slavery, and extreme trauma in psychoanalytic practice* (pp. 159–178). Routledge/Taylor & Francis Group.

Irving, D. (2014). *Waking up white: and finding myself in the story of race.* Elephant Room Press.

Kent, J. (2021) Scapegoating and the 'angry black woman. *Group Analysis, 54*(3), 354–371. https://doi.org/10.1177/0533316421992.

Layton, L. (2020). *Toward a social psychoanalysis: Culture, character, and normative unconscious processes.* (M. Leavy-Sperounis, Ed.). Routledge/Taylor & Francis Group.https://doi-org.fuller.idm.oclc.org/10.4324/9781003023098.

Leary, K. (2000). Racial enactments in dynamic treatment. *Psychoanalytic Dialogues, 10*(4), 639–653. https://doi.org/10.1080/10481881009348573.

Lee, M. W. (1994). *The color of fear.* StirFry Productions.

Lee, M. W. (2011). *Let's get real: What people of color can't say, and whites won't ask about racism.* StirFry Seminars & Consulting.

Lee, E., Tsang, A. K., Bogo, M., Johnstone, M., & Hershman, J. (2018). Enactments of racial microaggression in everyday therapeutic encounters. *Smith College Studies in Social Work, 88*(3), 211–236. https://doi.org/10.1080/00377317.2018.1476646.

Lefforge, N. L., McLaughlin, S., Goates-Jones, M., & Mejia, C. (2020). A training model for addressing microaggressions in group psychotherapy. *International Journal of Group Psychotherapy, 70*(1), 1–28. https://doi.org/10.1080/00207284.2019.1680989.

Miles, J. R., Anders, C., Kivlighan, D. M. III, & Belcher Platt, A. A. (2021). Cultural ruptures: Addressing microaggressions in group therapy. *Group Dynamics: Theory, Research, and Practice, 25*(1), 74–88. https://doi.org/10.1037/gdn0000149.

National Association of Social Workers. (2001, 2006, 2016). *Standards and indicators for cultural competence in Social Work Practice.* National Association of Social Workers, Washington, D.C.

Nayak, S. (2021). Black feminist intersectionality is vital to group analysis: Can group analysis allow outsider ideas in? *Group Analysis, 54*(3), 337–353. https://doi.org/10.1177/0533316421997.

Ortiz, L. & Jani, J. (2010). Critical race theory: A transformational model for teaching diversity. *Journal of Social Work Education, 46*(2), 175–193. https://doi.org/10.5175/JSWE.2010.200900070.

Powell, D. R. (2018). Race, African Americans, and psychoanalysis: Collective silence in the therapeutic situation. *Journal of the American Psychoanalytic Association, 66*(6), 1021–1049. https://doi.org/10.1177/0003065118818447.

Rutan, J. S. (2021). Rupture and repair: Using leader errors in psychodynamic group psychotherapy, *International Journal of Group Psychotherapy, 71*(2), 310–331. https://doi.org/10.1080/00207284.2020.1808471.

Schmidt, C. (2018). Anatomy of racial micro-aggressions. *International Journal of Group Psychotherapy, 68*(4), 585–607. DOI: 10.1080/00207284.2017.14214698.

Singh, A. A., Merchant, N., Skudrzyk, B., Ingene, D., Hutchins, A. M., & Rubel, D. (Collaborators). (2012). Association for specialists in group work: Multicultural and social justice competence principles for group workers. *Journal for Specialists in Group Work, 37*(4), 312–325. https://doi-org.fuller.idm.oclc.org/10.1080/01933922.2012.721482.

Stevenson, S. (2020). Psychodynamic intersectionality and the positionality of the group analyst: the tension between analytical neutrality and inter-subjectivity. *Group Analysis, 53*(4), 498–514. https://doi.org/10.1177/0533316420953660.

Sue, D. W., Capodilupo, C. M., Torino, G. C., Bucceri, J. M., Holder, A. M. B., Nadal, K. L., & Esquilin, M. (2007). Racial microaggressions in everyday life: Implications for clinical practice. *American Psychologist, 62*(4), 271–286. https://doi.org/10.1037/0003-066X.62.4.271.

Sue, D. W. (2015). *Race talk and the conspiracy of silence. Understanding and* facilitating difficult dialogues on race. John Wiley and Sons, Inc.

Tatum, B. D. (2017). *Why are all the Black kids sitting together in the cafeteria and other conversations about race, 2nd Edition.* Basic Books.

Tummala-Narra, P. (2016*). Psychoanalytic theory and cultural competence in psychotherapy.* American Psychological Association.

Yalom, I. D. & Leszcz, M. (2020). *The theory and practice of group psychotherapy.* Basic Books.

Yarborough, C. (2017). Being the only one: Finding connection through the shared experience of "otherness". *Smith College Studies in Social Work, 87*(2–3), 189–99. https://doi.org/10.1080/00377317.2017.1324078.

2 Addressing Power Dynamics in Systems-Centered Training Groups

Undoing Racialized Enactments by
Developing a Decolonizing Group Culture
and Weakening Closed Survivor-Roles

*Susan P. Gantt, Willard Ashley, Joan Adams,
and Frances Carter*

Our team of four (one Black woman, one Black man, and two White women) has drawn from the conceptual frames of Systems-Centered Training and Therapy (SCT) and its theory of living human systems (TLHS)[1] (Agazarian, 1997) and from the field of anti-racism (Ashley, 2021) in exploring how to address racialized power dynamics in SCT training groups. We have concluded that it is imperative to train group leaders in both sensitivity to racism and recognition of the implicit level at which all groups enact racialized dynamics, stimulated both by group phases of development and our larger cultural and historical contexts. Group dynamics embody and reveal racism, so that didactic education alone will never be enough to change racist dynamics: this requires experiential learning to recognize, explore, and modify racialized enactments fueled by and embodied by group dynamics so that groups can develop decolonizing cultures rather than perpetuating racism.

Although becoming knowledgeable about racialized trauma, racism, and anti-racism is essential for group therapists, it is not enough to support sustained change. As Menakem (2017) writes: "We've tried to teach our brains to think better about race. But white-body supremacy doesn't live in our thinking brains. It lives and breathes in our bodies" (p. 5). As group therapists, we know that sustained change comes from new experiences with others in groups that both introduce differences to us and support us as human beings in integrating new and different experiences. Group therapy can change our neurobiology, both our embodied nervous system and our brains (Flores, 2010; Gantt, 2018, 2019; Gantt & Agazarian, 2010), increasing our capacity to explore dynamics and differences. Lastly, we know that when groups fixate by enacting group dynamics or reacting to differences, new experiences cannot be integrated.

From the lens of SCT and its TLHS, sustainable change necessitates changes in both structure and function for all living human systems. Viewed from TLHS, changing laws alters structure. For example, the US Supreme Court ruled in 1954 against racial segregation in public schools. Despite this legal structure, the ruling has not **yet** enabled the function and norms to fully change 70 years later. Changing norms requires not only changing **both** structure and function in a living human system but also weakening the restraining forces such as racism that maintain systems in survival at the expense of development and transformation (Agazarian, 1997). Living human systems *function* to survive, develop and transform through the process of identifying or discriminating differences so differences can be

DOI: 10.4324/9781003455783-4

explored and integrated.[2] Closing our boundaries to differences supports survival of "what is" at the expense of development and change.

Given 1) the pervasiveness of both explicit and implicit racism (structural and functional) in the US; and 2) that training groups exist within this cultural context, we assume that training groups will inevitably enact racist dynamics in the authority phase of group development where group dynamics relate to power and control (Agazarian, 1997). Authority phase group dynamics stimulate closed survivor-roles related to power and control (Gantt et al., 2021). SCT defines closed survivor-roles as subsystems in a person which develop in response to affiliation/attachment or socializing challenges (Gantt, 2021). These closed survivor-roles (especially those related to socialization) easily enact and sustain the same racialized group dynamics which exist in the world. We will describe how the group dynamics aroused in the authority phase are embodied in specific closed survivor-roles, the structure of which functions to maintain racist power dynamics. We underscore the imperative for experiential group training in which these authority phase dynamics are explored so that group therapists learn to weaken their closed survivor-roles so that the racialized dynamics can be explored in the context of group development, facilitating a group that is freer to explore and weaken racism in its here-and-now context.

Conceptual Frame: The Theory Behind SCT

SCT's TLHS defines a hierarchy of isomorphic systems that are energy-organizing, goal-directing, and self-correcting (Agazarian, 1997). Isomorphy means similarity in structure and function for systems in a nested hierarchy. Hierarchy defines that a system always exists within the context of a larger system, and the system itself is the context of the system below it in the hierarchy (Figure 2.1). There is an infinite hierarchy of isomorphic living human systems, yet SCT always works with the set of three nested systems that are most relevant to the goal and context.

Seeing all living human systems as a hierarchy of three isomorphic systems helps us recognize how larger system norms govern smaller systems that exist within the larger system context (Figure 2.2). Systems govern people. Realizing that how we function has more to do with system norms than just our person system resources lowers our human pull to personalize. The middle system in the hierarchy (Figure 2.2) is the most influential for system change as it sets norms that govern the system below it in the hierarchy and directly influences the system above it. Operationally defining system hierarchy has led to SCT's emphasis on contextualizing as an antidote to personalizing.

Person system energy (Figure 2.3) fuels all hierarchies of living human systems. Each system in the hierarchy organizes this energy toward implicit and explicit goals. Thinking

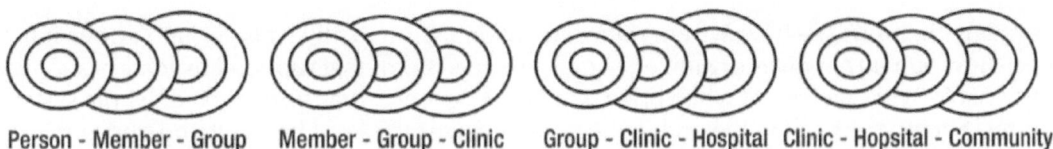

Person - Member - Group   Member - Group - Clinic   Group - Clinic - Hospital   Clinic - Hopsital - Community

Figure 2.1 Infinite hierarchy of isomorphic systems.

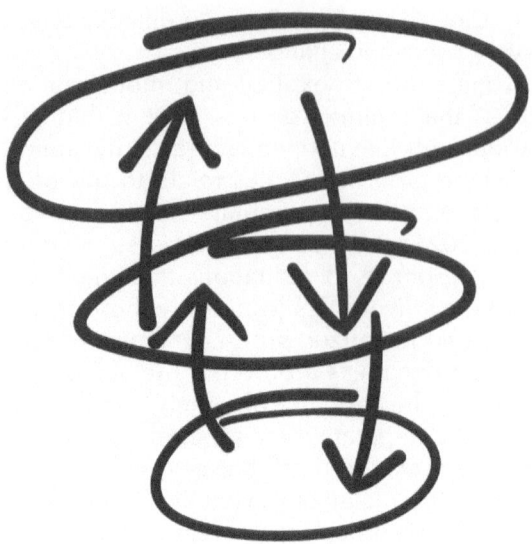

Figure 2.2 System is influenced by the system above it in the hierarchy and influences the system below it.

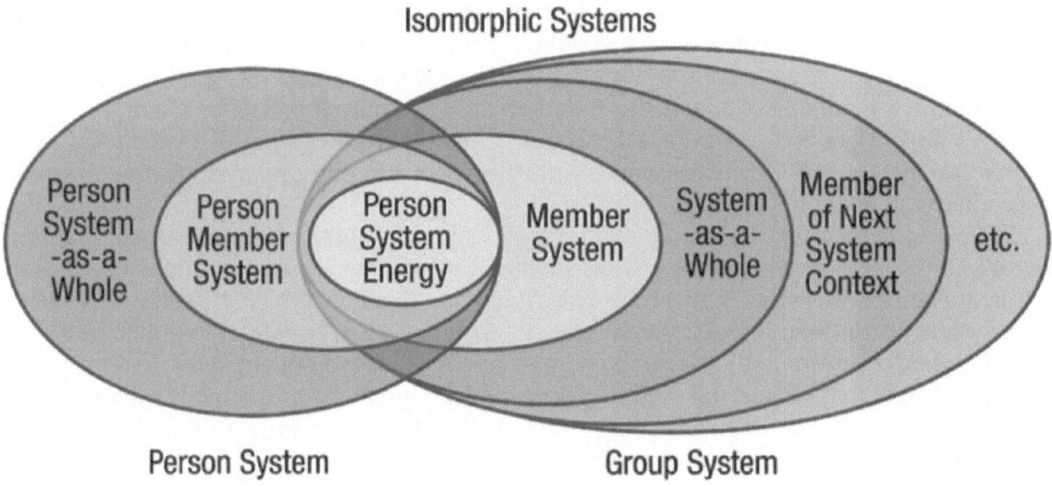

Figure 2.3 Person system energy fuels all system levels.

"systems" helps us see how system norms maintain racism at all levels. System norms influence how human energy is organized in closed role-systems that support the goals of *survival* of "what is," e.g., racism, or when open, the *development* or *transformation* of whole system norms. Each system in the hierarchy directly influences the level below it and above it.

We can define a system hierarchy (Figure 2.4) for conceptualizing racism in the US, e.g., our person-as-a-whole system nested in our family-systems-as-a-whole, which are nested in our country-as-a-whole. In this hierarchy, the family-system and its norms have the most influence, as the middle system directly influences the system above it and below it.

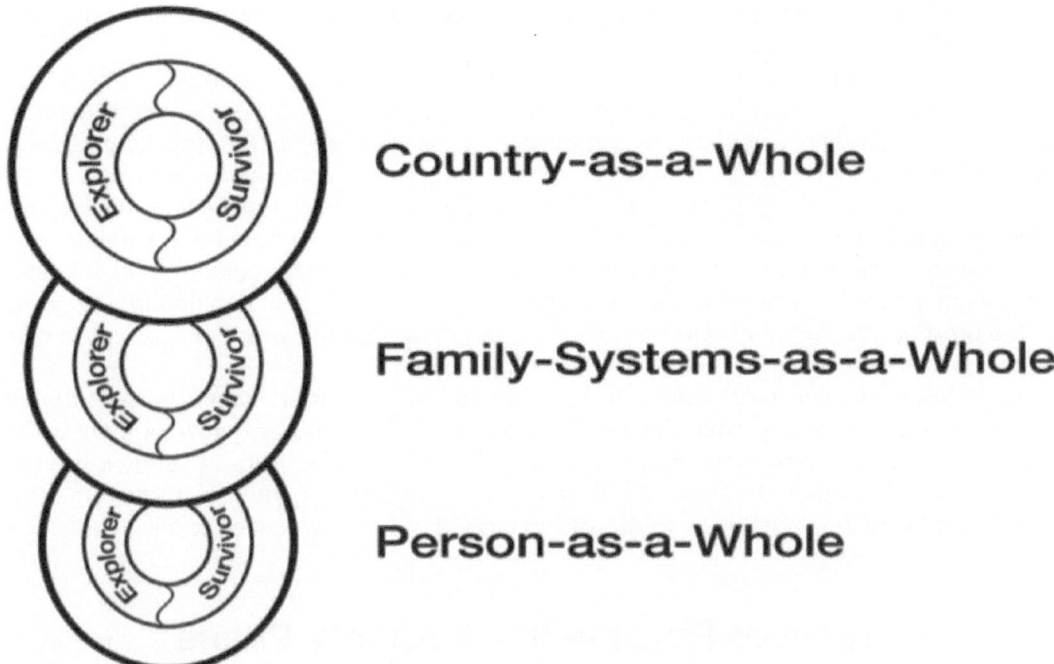

Country-as-a-Whole

Family-Systems-as-a-Whole

Person-as-a-Whole

Figure 2.4 All systems at all levels of the hierarchy have both survivor- and explorer-roles.

Our inner-person (center circle in each hierarchy in Figure 2.4) contains the person system energy for all living human systems (Figure 2.3). We have two role-systems (explorer-role and survivor-role) that first develop in our inner-person system. Iterations of these role-systems exist at all levels of the hierarchy. In our explorer-role, we have curiosity, signaling open boundaries and potential for development. In our closed survivor-roles, our major goal is survival, stability, and staying with what we know.

All hierarchies of systems have both potentials for organizing energy: in explorer- or survivor-roles at any system level. Survivor-roles orient to the known and explorer-roles open to the unknown. The developmental phase of the larger system in any system hierarchy influences all the systems in the nested hierarchy, its phase dynamics, and implicit and explicit norms. SCT posits that who we are and how we behave has as much or more to do with the system we are in and the group's phase than with ourselves and our person system dynamics (Agazarian & Gantt, 2003).

Seeing Racism Through the Lens of SCT Theory

The authority phase is dominant in our country-as-a-system. Its major dynamics relate to *power and control*, and contain the subphases of flight, fight, roles/role-locks, and the crisis of hatred (Agazarian, 1997). A widely used definition of racism is prejudice linked with *power and control*. Applying SCT theory, the issues of racism are most pervasive in the authority phase. Given our historical context and our larger system norms supporting racism, the survivor-roles that we enact in the authority phase will reflect colonization and

racism, with our closed survivor-roles of compliance in the flight subphase and our dominant or submissive survivor-roles in the fight subphase.

Racism can then be defined by the output of the system, e.g., country-as-a-system in
the authority phase, where the dynamics related to power and control are fueled by prejudice. Using SCT theory, we can hypothesize that the authority phase and its prototypic
survivor-roles are the group dynamic iteration of racist structure and function within a
person-as-a-system, a family-as-a-system, or our country-as-a-system. Testing this requires
identifying racism in our whole system context and assessing how our closed survivor-roles
and role-locks enact racialized pairings that maintain a colonizing culture at each system
level (Figure 2.5). Our closed survivor-roles reflect past adaptations and maintain past norms
in the present. We are all puppets on the strings of the phase dynamics of our system contexts unless we are actively undoing our closed survivor-roles.

Our closed survivor-roles' outputs enact and maintain the phase dynamics, contributing
to the stability of what is and has been in terms of racism. This sabotages development which
can only happen by first weakening the restraining forces in our closed survivor-roles so
that our roles can open to differences, develop, and transform, enabling our role outputs to
contribute to creating a pathway for transformation of our whole system norms.

Survivor-Roles in the Authority Phase

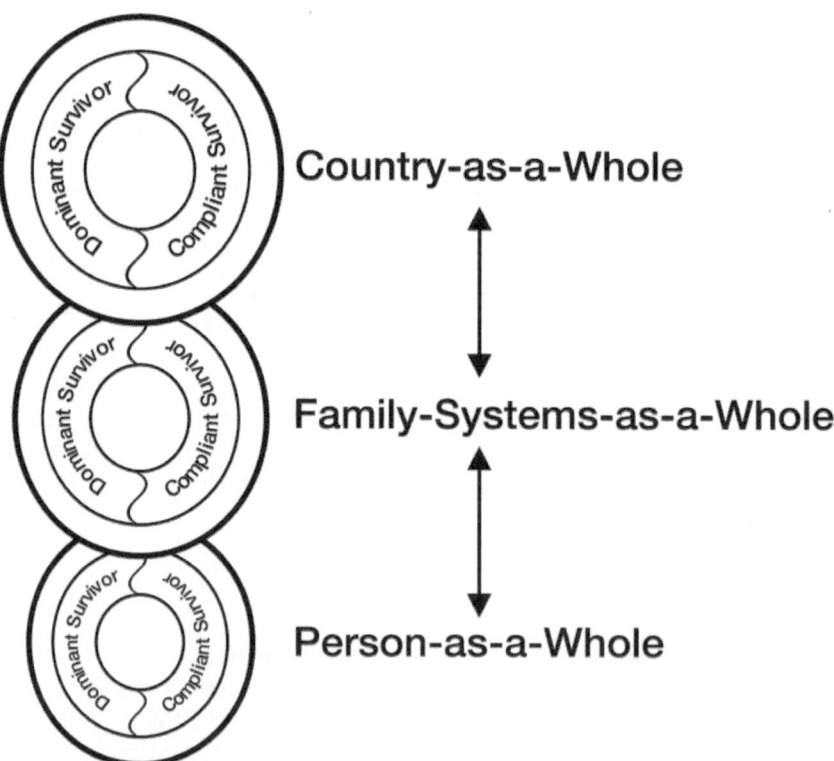

Figure 2.5 Survivor-roles in the authority phase.

All of us have survivor-role adaptations (Ashley et al., 2022). Our racialized closed survivor-role adaptations relate to racialized experiences in our families and communities and are inevitably reenacted in the context of group dynamics. Training groups are a unique opportunity for seeing our racialized survivor-roles in the context of authority phase power dynamics. As group trainers, recognizing these role enactments and their racialized contexts enables us to support the group doing the developmental role work that makes it possible to have different discussions about race and racism. Without this developmental work, all of us will continue to enact our closed survivor-roles, maintaining racism and its denial. For group trainers, recognizing our own closed survivor-roles and those of our group members is imperative if we are to courageously embrace racialized conflicts (Ashley, 2021) and *explore* the survivor-role adaptations as they emerge in our groups rather than smoothing them over or legislating "proper" behavior. Though not easy, it is vital in training group leaders that we provide group experiences in which racialized dynamics can be explored as they emerge within the group dynamics in each developmental phase, different from teaching members nonracist or politically correct behaviors.

Recognizing how implicit racism is maintained by the interplay of group dynamics and closed survivor-roles is essential for group leaders. Taking these understandings to heart, experiential group training can explore implicit and explicit expressions of racism, enabling us to discover how our closed survivor-role adaptations maintain the status quo. Failing to see our closed survivor-roles in the context of power and control (an essential component of racism and the heart of the authority phase) leads to reiterating the functional and structural racism that group dynamics do enact and maintain. As group therapists, we are uniquely qualified to do this work, making it an ethical imperative for us to do so.

SCT Theory into Practice: Group Interventions

SCT's methods (contextualizing, functional subgrouping, boundarying, vectoring) put its theory into practice to develop collaborative and decolonizing contexts. *Contextualizing* teaches groups to see themselves and others in the context of system hierarchies which normalizes, legitimizes, humanizes, contextualizes, and de-pathologizes all human experience and behavior. Contextualizing lowers personalizing. Personalizing closes our boundaries to differences. Contextualizing also enables seeing our closed survivor-role adaptations in our historical, societal context with its past and current racist structures and implicit norms. Closed survivor-roles are transmitted generationally, and have adaptive value originally, yet they contain role outputs that maintain historical norms and stability at the expense of developing new norms in the present. These closed roles imprison us and others into replicating and maintaining what was. SCT's concept of closed-boundary survivor-roles is reminiscent of the analytic concept of the repetition compulsion where early life experiences or adaptations are reenacted.

SCT groups use *functional subgrouping* (FSG), exploring with others who feel similarly as an alternative to reacting to differences. Each difference is explored in a separate subgroup until the differences can be integrated. *Boundarying* orients to observing when our boundaries are open or closed and, over time, learning to titrate the permeability of system boundaries as we explore our closed racialized survivor-roles. Both of these methods enable groups to modify communications by building a base for recognizing and undoing our inevitable here-and-now closed-boundary survivor-role outputs (both verbal and non-verbal behaviors) that maintain past racist norms and stereotypic hierarchies. For example, lengthy explaining is often flight into verbal dominance and away from making space to explore new or different information in the present.

Vectoring orients to noticing the implicit goal of how our energy is organized, e.g., staying the same (enacting closed survivor-roles) or exploring our experience in the present (explorer-role). By identifying "forks-in-the-road," groups learn to deliberately choose what to explore in each phase-specific dynamic. For example, in the flight subphase, groups learn the difference between explaining (flight) or exploring their experience. In the fight subphase, SCT introduces the "fork-in-the-road" between exploring the impulse to enact or exploring the experience that the enactment discharges.

Closed survivor-roles stabilize "what is." Open survivor- and explorer-roles support integrating differences. Integrating differences is the process by which all living human systems survive, develop, and transform from simpler to more complex living human systems with greater resources for solving the conflicts inherent in system development and transformation. Theoretically, closed survivor-roles can be operationally defined by the properties of all living human systems (Agazarian et al., 2021): context, boundaries open or closed, capacity for discriminating and integrating differences, and goal orientation (survival, development, or transformation).

Applying TLHS in the context of racial trauma, all of us have developed closed survivor-roles in our earlier and ongoing racialized contexts to adapt, with White people frequently in dominating, "head-in-the-sand" or spectator roles with dissociation or care-taking. People of Color often adapt by scanning for danger, with survivor-roles of compliant, dissociative, defiant, or submissive. If not weakened and explored, these roles fixate the group and members in flight/fight patterns replicating past racialized hierarchies.

In the authority phase, groups avoid differences by ignoring (flight) or scapegoating them (fight) by attacking, criticizing, or trying to convert differences. As Finlay et al. (2016) suggested: scapegoating is a "communal survival tactic." We would add that scapegoating is the output of a closed-boundary "fight" survivor-role, keeping differences out and maintaining what is. Similarly, "avoiding" signals a closed "flight" survivor-role, ignoring or not seeing differences. All closed survivor-roles, flight or fight, orient to the goal of survival and stability by closing boundaries to differences. Closed survivor-roles fixate in survival, maintaining stability at all system levels at the expense of integrating differences which are essential for development.

Building a Decolonizing Group: Functional Subgrouping (FSG) as an Antidote to Enacting Racism by Splitting and Extruding Differences and Creating Identified-Patients or Scapegoats

Differences are essential for development, yet opening our boundaries to differences is destabilizing (Agazarian, 1997). FSG enables shifting out of stereotyping gender, race or culture to exploring the actual similarities and differences in race, culture and gender in our here-and-now experience so that the differences can be integrated as resources for the group's (and members') development (Gantt & Adams, 2010) rather than avoided or scapegoated. Exploring here-and-now experience about racism makes it less likely that education unwittingly enacts the power dynamics that fuel racism and which easily induces racialized enactments in compliance or sabotage, at the expense of exploring the racialized power dynamics fueling compliance or sabotage.

By establishing FSG as a norm, no member works alone. Each member's input is seen as a voice for a subgroup in the group, not just "personal" to the person. Group members first *reflect* the heart of what the other person has said until they feel understood, and then *add* something that is similar. In establishing the norm of FSG, SCT leaders interrupt "yes, but" communications which close boundaries to differences, e.g., "but" discounts and dismisses the "yes." Instead FSG requires that someone reflect and build on the previous contribution before checking to see if the group is ready for a difference (Agazarian et al., 2021). Closing boundaries to differences sabotages the group's development. For example (Figure 2.5), in an anti-racism study group where the pattern of FSG was not yet a norm, a Black member brought in his despair ("this organization will never really change") and his impulse to leave rather than "go along." A White member reacted: explaining how it wasn't so bad. This implicit "yes, but" communication from her closed survivor-role dropped him and the depth of his feeling.

Through the SCT lens, the White member went into a care-taking survivor-role and the Black member "went along" by staying silent, resulting in his despair being minimized. FSG requires shifting out of the "yes, but" pattern to form two subgroups, in this example: 1) those resonating with a "going-along" role exploring together; and 2) those noticing their "care-taking" role exploring together. This enables exploration of both survivor-roles in a context of similarity where small differences could be integrated and the roles (and ultimately the group) could develop by discriminating and integrating the differences. Later in this group's development, e.g., in the intimacy phase, the work might be more focused on the alienation and despair of never being understood or acknowledged.

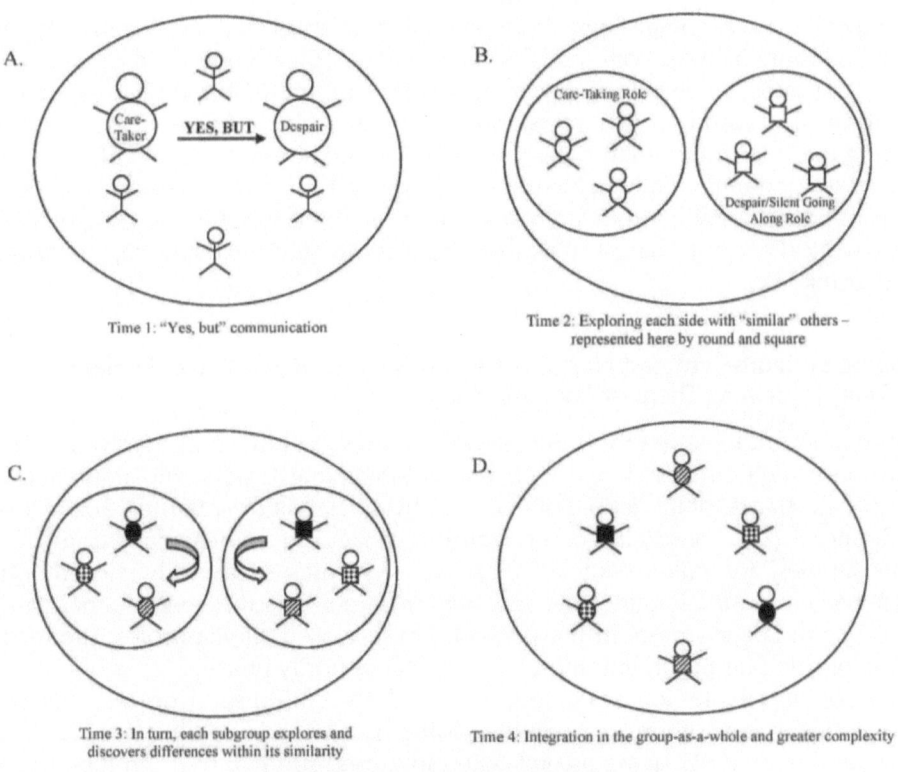

© S.P. Gantt, 2023. Adapted from Agazarian, 1997.

Figure 2.6 Functional subgrouping: Integrating similarities and differences.

SCT groups establish FSG as a group norm immediately before the group imports stereotypic social norms which reinforce survivor-roles. With FSG as a norm, no one holds a difference alone. Instead, each difference is explored in a subgroup with those who share the difference until the differences can be integrated rather than avoided (flight) or scapegoated (fight). FSG implements a TLHS: living human systems develop and transform by discriminating and integrating differences, differences in the apparently similar and similarities in the initially different (Agazarian, 1997). FSG creates containment by establishing a climate of coregulation (Gantt, 2018, 2019) where boundaries open more easily to differences as an alternative to the activation of our closed-boundary survivor-roles where boundaries closed to differences maintain the status quo. Importantly, FSG lowers the scapegoating of differences that is endemic in racism in the authority phase given our racialized culture.

Modifying Role-System Outputs to Influence Survivor-Roles

Once FSG is established as a group norm, the group has a containing context to modify the survivor-role outputs relevant in each phase of group development. For example, in the flight subphase communications are vague and ambiguous to avoid differences, stay safe and not "rock the boat." Weakening these flight communication patterns introduces differences yet when done in the context of subgrouping, the difference is easier to integrate, e.g., when several members are ambiguous, the leader suggests they subgroup together to be more specific. Weakening "flight" from differences enables the group's transition into fight, where the communication pattern shifts to "yes, but." SCT works with "yes, but" as two different subgroups, as described earlier. Over time, by modifying the role-system outputs and exploring the closed survivor-roles, the roles open to small differences, the beginning of *developing* the roles rather than *reiterating* them. In the authority phase, SCT first modifies the role-system outputs in the flight subphase, then in turn, fight, roles and role-locks, and the crisis of hatred, moving from simpler work in the flight subphase to progressively more complex work. Each subphase builds the resources for the next subphase conflicts to be explored using FSG.

Developing Systems-Centered Norms for Exploring Racialized Power Dynamics Rather Than Explaining Them or Enacting Them

Inevitably in group therapy today, the power dynamics will have isomorphic (similarity in structure and function) resonance with our colonializing history and traumatic survivor adaptations of Blacks, other People of Color and Whites (Major & Barndt, 2023; Menakem, 2017; Stoute, 2023). These closed survivor-roles enact our earlier adaptations, reiterating both our families' and culture's racialized power dynamics, structurally (closed boundaries to differences) and functionally (scapegoating or care-taking differences), maintaining our countries' colonializing pasts in the present. These closed survivor-roles often surface as role-locks or role-pairings in training groups in the authority phase.

The rest of this chapter focuses on our work with the closed survivor-roles that emerge in training groups in the authority phase: describing how we are working with the isomorphy of racism in the authority phase as embodied in closed survivor-roles (in the inner-person) and role-locks of identified-patient/helper, one-up/one-down, dominant/submissive or subjugated, and defiant/compliant that maintain colonization patterns at the inter-person (member) and whole-system levels.

Case Examples

We have included three case examples from different SCT contexts for training group leaders. Our first example describes how we "discovered" the relationship between group dynamics and racism that enabled us to recognize how the authority phase dynamics enact and maintain racism. Though obvious to us now, it was only in watching the group and its phase-specific survivor-roles that we clearly saw the interface between racism and the group dynamics in the authority phase. This recognition spawned our commitment to explore how group dynamics maintain and enact racism. Our second and third examples illustrate how we have been applying our "discovery" in training SCT group leaders about the inevitable interface between group dynamics, closed survivor-roles, and racism.

Discovering How Group Dynamics and Racism Are Intertwined

In a two-day SCT large group, the early phase flight dynamics were being enacted by the group implicitly electing two women of Color into the role of "identified-patients" who were then "helped" or "taken care of" by two White men. This was initially quite subtle, yet as the interactions continued, the care-taking became more pronounced as a White European male repeatedly checked his mindreads (e.g., assumptions) with a BIPOC female who became increasingly uncomfortable with the repetition:

White male:	My mindread is that you are uncomfortable in this group?
BIPOC female:	No
Leader:	Do you believe her?
White male:	Yes
Leader:	Are you curious, since you believe her, how your mindread might be a projection[3] since it is not a perception?

His mindreads were outputs from a closed survivor-role. This was early in our first meeting, and the group had not yet developed its resources to work directly with undoing the implicit role-lock that was emerging. In undoing his mindread, he was shifting from a closed survivor-role to a curious explorer-role which contributed to the group's developing reality-testing. Weakening the flight enactments into speculative thoughts built a reality-testing culture, essential work in the flight phase.

SCT leaders deliberately establish the norm of reality-testing, both by undoing negative predictions about the future and mindreads of others in the present. For example, a member voiced: "I don't think I am going to like this group." Undoing this by reality-testing the negative prediction enabled the group to work in the present rather than in speculation or predictions about the future. When SCT groups undo mindreads, the group also strengthens its reality-testing culture in the here-and-now. Both skills are introduced in the flight subphase, enabling the group to weaken the flight into speculation and opinion and away from the here-and-now.

Once reality-testing was established in this group, the leader named the implicit roles (care-taking and identified-patient) signaled by the redundant negative predictions and mindreads and framed this role-pairing as two subgroups for the group to explore.

The identified-patient subgroup explored how they wanted the group to "help" them. The other subgroup explored how they wanted to "take care of" the identified-patients, either trying to be helpful or "taking care" of the problem by getting rid of the difference the identified-patients were voicing. Exploring these flight roles weakened their implicit one-up/one-down role patterns.

Freed from these flight roles, tension then emerged in the group. Tension blocks access to our emotional knowing, and surfaces in the transition from flight to fight. Weakening tension restores a primary relationship to our emotional and bodily knowing. The leaders guided the tension[4] subgroup in either melting their tension to free their experience or living inside the tension to discover what experience was being blocked, providing this structure for the subgroup to use in undoing their bodily tension. In SCT, this work is an essential step in the process of restoring our relationship with our bodies,[5] vital in working with racial trauma and dissociation.

In the next group sessions, free from tension and with greater access to emotions, a subgroup explored first frustration, then anger, and then the hatred of the group leaders as the stand-in for all authorities who let us down and oppress us. In this process, the subgroup connected deeply with their own power and free aggression, feeling new, freer energy in their bodies and great pleasure with images emerging of destroying the leaders and gaining freedom from tyranny. They felt free and powerful in hating the leader and exploring their sadistic impulses toward the leader. Another subgroup noticed they had closed their boundaries, dissociating, or disconnecting during the exploration of hatred and the images of torturing the leaders. This subgroup then worked together exploring their tendency to cut off emotional knowing as an old way of surviving and in doing so felt sad for themselves which restored their connection to themselves again and to others in their subgroup.[6]

All of this work developed the group's resources for working together with the earlier racialized mindreads. Free of the avoidance of flight enacted by the White male projecting into the Black female and of the sadistic/masochistic roles in fight, the group was then able to explore and discover that some members felt their boundaries had been more closed to the People of Color in the group and others more open. The group felt and voiced the importance of the step they had made, in developing as a group and then being able to address the reactions to racial differences in the here-and-now with curiosity rather than enacting familiar survivor-roles. Initially the flight survivor-roles enacted in the role-lock between the Black woman and White man stabilized the whole group system in a replication of survivor norms with racist roots at the expense of exploring the here-and-now realities and challenges of racism.

This group enabled us to understand how racist dynamics are fueled by the authority phase in both flight and fight and its enactments around power and control, e.g., the White male enacted the one-up care-taking role and tried to induce the Black woman into one-down so he could "take care" of her. This led us to recognize that working with the authority phase dynamics is an essential context for undoing these phase survivor-roles that enact the implicit power dynamics that maintain racism. Seeing this led us to understand how essential this work is in training group leaders. Modifying the phase-specific restraining forces not only potentiated the group's development (which we expected), but also (surprisingly) undid the racialized role-lock enactments and freed resources for conversations in the group that earlier in the group not been possible. By weakening the flight and fight roles, the group could then rely on the containment that FSG provided to explore their sadistic hatred of authority. This led us to hypothesize that influencing system development by undoing the prototypic closed survivor-roles in each subphase of the authority phase enables groups to explore and weaken the here-and-now enactment of racist dynamics. These dynamics are embedded in not only our societal structures and laws but also in the norms of U.S. culture, our interactions in everyday life, and manifested in group dynamics.[7]

We all developed closed survivor-roles as adaptations to our family and cultural contexts. From this example, we hypothesized that "taking care of" People of Color [both meanings of "taking care of": helping ("there, there, don't worry" in the flight subphase) and scape-goating in the fight subphase (taking care of differences in the way the Mafia does it: "I will take care of you") have generational roots in role-pairings of slave owners and slaves. The reciprocal roles of identified-patient (or rebel) likely enabled many slaves to survive the dominance and sadism of the slave owners. Generational transmission of these roles continued these implicit survivor norms that sustain colonization patterns in everyday interactions and certainly in both training and therapy groups. Seeing how these role-pairings enabled survival at many levels helps us operationally define how our survivor-role outputs sustain the very norms that govern us and others. As system norms govern people, it is imperative to explore how our past adaptive survivor-roles maintain racist system norms that imprison all of us in closed survivor-roles.

By seeing group dynamics from our colonialized context, group leaders can support the group's exploration of authority phase survivor-roles (identified-patient/helper, one-up/one-down, dominant/submissive, defiant/compliant, bully/victim, sadistic/masochistic) as they emerge in the group. Weakening these survivor-roles frees the group to explore its hatred of authority rather than stabilizing in survivor-roles.

Exploring hatred toward the leader transformed this group from fixating in traumatic reen-actments and closed survivor-roles that defended against the sadism. This is essential work in training group leaders if we are to weaken the racialized enactments. Free of the bondage of closed survivor-roles, this group (Whites, Blacks and People of Color) bonded together to explore their murderous and sadistic impulses toward the leaders, the stand-in for all who had failed them. Bonding together and discovering and experiencing the depths of human hatred transformed the group into potency and gratitude toward the leaders for containing their depth of free experience. And most importantly, the group then returned to the earlier "denied" racism and acknowledged its reality. This transformation is similar to what de Maré called "the impersonal fellowship of Koinonia" (de Maré et al., 1991, p. 4) which we propose begins to lay an alternative pathway to the:

> . . . dominance hierarchies . . . established by the Europeans who colonized Africa and transported enslaved Africans. . . . The slave trade established a racialized hierarchy of social groupings . . . [and our racialized hierarchy of groupings prevented hatred from being metabolized and allowed racialized destructiveness] . . . against those of African descent, as racial objects become the allowable objects of sadistic destructiveness rather than developing a sense of guilt . . . unbound destructive power and sadism was then passed down to the next generation. This sadism is enjoyed, the hate goes on unmetabo-lized, and is enacted. . . . We are blind to racial enactments . . . in not seeing we are remembering in action, we do not have verbal access to the preverbal racial memory that is being put into action.
>
> (Stoute, 2022)

Our discoveries from this group fueled our determination to explore more deeply how SCT groups can weaken racialized role enactments and role-locks (in this example, helper/identified-patient) that maintain racism by "remembering in action." When this group had weakened their roles and role-locks with each other, they were free to explore together their impulses, feelings and fantasized "actions" in the containment of the subgrouping and the leader. The emergent sadism and hatred toward the authority as the symbol of oppression, and which the racialized survivor-roles had both enacted and defended from experiencing, were then transformed into free energy and power.

In this group, "remembering in action" was apparent in the early phase survivor-role enactments which were implicitly racialized. Undoing the two survivor-roles through the subgrouping exploration opened the pathway for exploring sadism, masochism and hatred rather than enacting it destructively in closed survivor-roles that maintained racialized adaptations. Exploration in FSG with the leaders as the target contained the racial hatred and enabled the free energy in hatred to be accessed and integrated rather than enacted in survivor-roles that maintain enactments of the racialized sadistic destructiveness that is then passed on generationally. Building on this discovery, the four of us worked together to apply these learnings in our yearly SCT training conference.

Our Next Steps: Training Group Therapists and Consultants

In our SCT conference-as-a-whole workshop (100+ people), "Working with Systemic Racism and Its Impact" (Ashley et al., 2022), Ashley first introduced anti-racist theory, drawing from Tuzzolo's triangle [2016; adapted from Safehouse Progressive Alliance for Nonviolence, 2005] (EmbraceRace, 2020). The smaller apex of the triangle lists the *socially unacceptable* signs of overt White Supremacy culture that are easily prohibited: "hate crimes, lynching, racial slurs, violence, inappropriate language, and symbols with harmful racial history." Below the apex, the larger area of the triangle, are the *"socially accepted* forms of racist behaviors: denial of racism; mass incarceration; racial profiling; paternalism, school-to-prison pipeline; police brutality; discriminatory lending; Euro-centered education; denial of White privilege; self-appointed White ally; claims of reverse racism; unjustified fear of People of Color; banning materials which describe slavery, violent acts against Black people or Black history/culture; tokenism; exceptionalism; color blindness and the rugged individualism bootstrap theory", which are harmful when racist myths, distortions, and lies go unchecked or unchallenged.

Following this orientation, we summarized SCT's theory on how phase-specific survivor-roles maintain racism and racialized enactments. Building from our hypothesis that undoing survivor-roles lowers racist enactments in the authority phase, we introduced a modification of SCT's role protocol (Agazarian et al., 2021) that enabled seeing our survivor roles with an explicit awareness of their roots in the context of racism.

We first demonstrated the exercise described below and then randomly assigned members to small triads to do the work together.

Triad Instructions:[8]

Pick a survivor-role to explore today: a Flight role (Helper or Identified-Patient) or a Fight role (Compliant or Defiant).

As you join your triad, remember to build on each other as you explore together, going through the questions together and making time for each person's answer.

1. Tell your group which role you picked to explore today, give your role a personal name.
2. In this role, what were your boundaries open to today? What have your boundaries closed to today? Tell each other.

3. Thinking about system hierarchy, identify from your family of origin, your family system's flight or fight role in the context of racism [was it closer to a Flight role (Helper, Identified-Patient) or a Fight role (Compliant or Defiant)?]. Tell each other.
4. Give a personal name to your family's flight or fight role. Tell each other.
5. Identify a driving force and/or a restraining force in your family's role in how this role contributed to the larger system norms in the context of racism. Tell each other.
6. What is it like for you now to see your family's role in the context of racism? Tell each other.
7. What is it like to see your flight or fight role in this group after looking at your family's role? Tell each other.
8. Say Goodbye to your group in your last 2 minutes.

Following the exercise, the whole large group[9] shared Surprises, Learnings, Satisfactions, Dissatisfactions and Discoveries[10] (SLSDD) from their triad work. A sample of these are included here:

Surprised and satisfied to learn how clueless I am in my family system about my race, power, activeness, and passivity and internalized racism.

Learning in my triad that my family of origin was in fight and defiance, and I'm in that as well. Cost is that I have not explored my compliant roles: "Don't rock the boat" or "Just let it go," "You're not going to make a difference." I discovered I have a lot of disgust for those roles.

Discovered the name of my role is "special White person," and that goes both for the fight energy in naming some racism but also from staying "one-up."

Discovered how a "nice guy" role can be a very closed survival role. "Nice guy" knows all the stuff in the apex of the pyramid and doesn't put up with it. "Total oblivion" in most of my life to what's below it.

Relearning when I'm in a group of White people, I don't feel White. And when I'm in a group of People of Color, I feel very White. My identity is relative. Also surprised how much fight I felt during this workshop, and aware of how much fight I almost always have.

Being brought up Jewish with strong annihilation fears, I am so surprised how my family had strong compliance and a desire for one-up, that those things existed together, that they couldn't see beyond their own fears and so were deeply racist and taught us too. Also noticed my choosing a helper role, that had defiance in it, not just compliance.

My family system escaping Nazi Germany as Jews and the sense that when we came to this country, we really just poured ourselves in as immigrants. Learning how we just put blinders on and ignored everything else and just focused on our own survival in my family.

Discovery about intergenerational transfer of racism in my family and how it's gone from being overt and just becoming more covert down the generations. I need to find out where it's hiding in me.

Our Third Example

One year later, again at our SCT training conference for group leaders, three of us presented the conference-as-a-whole closing workshop focused on leading edges in SCT and entitled "Whatever We Say a Thing Isn't, It IS!" (Adams et al., 2023). This was the last event in a seven-day training conference so almost all participants had some prior experience with SCT training, be it during the preceding week or previously.

We first summarized racism in the US and then described using SCT theory as a lens for seeing how survivor-roles maintain systemic racism (Gantt et al., 2021). Participants then viewed a live role-play of a White therapist with a Black client, the therapist enacting a dominant survivor-role while undoing anxiety[11] with the client, and then a second White therapist role-playing a compliant survivor-role while undoing anxiety with the same Black client. There were strong emotions as the 90+ people present watched, feeling the harm that was apparent even though we all knew the demonstrations were role-plays.

We then introduced an exercise where participants worked in small groups taking turns role-playing closed survivor-roles while implementing SCT's protocol for undoing anxiety as they had just observed. This exercise was especially important to us, as SCT group leaders regularly introduce significant structure to enable members and subgroups to find alternative forks to closed survivor-roles. Not surprisingly, holding tight structures can easily stimulate the authority issue when the structure is applied from a compliant or dominant survivor role without attunement to the person and their context. We designed the exercise to increase sensitivity to how leaders enact closed survivor-roles with racist overtones.

We had not anticipated that asking participants to experience themselves in the roles that they had observed arousing such strong emotions would stimulate authority issues and closed survivor-roles with us as the workshop leaders (one Black woman and two White women). We were struck by the isomorphy (that what we were asking them to do stimulated their authority role-locks with us) as we were asking them to experiment with enacting a closed survivor authority role in the exercises.

We implemented the exercise by dividing the large group into triads to work with the same protocol for undoing anxiety that they had observed and asking them to alternate role-playing using the protocol from either a dominant or compliant survivor-role with an observer watching what happened. The experience was sobering for all, and especially for the majority of attendees, White therapists, coaches, and leaders who saw how easily they participated in enacting and maintaining a racist power dynamic irrespective of the client's color. Several of the SLSDD are below:

> We were surprised at the potential sadism in the protocol itself if it's implemented in a dominant way.

> Surprised how quickly when I joined a White-only triad, I dropped race as part of it, thinking it's just White people so it's not about race.

> We also felt it was hard, it created a lot more induction and insecurity, actually increased anxiety and we became more authoritarian.

> Learning that when leading from a dominant survivor-role, my client lost everything they knew, and I could see them looking for themselves everywhere else than themselves.

> We discovered our dominant position induced a reciprocal dominant role in the client.

A big learning being the client with a submissive therapist who just wanted to please, be nice to me and help me, and didn't give me enough structure. How unhelpful that was, he would probably not understand why I didn't like him because he was trying so hard to be helpful.

Discovered sadism in the compliant role, abandoning and leaving it all up to the client to do the work.

In observer role, watching a dominant leader and discovered the phrase, "just following orders" bubble up in me followed by disgust.

With the compliant therapist, the client went from aggression and anger to feeling sick. That parallels Black people having more medical sickness. White compliance contributes that to our system, making people sick, Black people sick, and negating the aggression.

I discovered some scapegoating tendency in us, in our group.

Deep satisfaction: I feel surprised at being much more aware of both of my roles that I enact with clients, and curious if I take this with me. It's not what I want to do, but it's making me more sensitive.

Discovered when I'm with a White client, I can easily do these two positions of dominant and submissive, and as soon as I realized I was having a client of Color, a Black client in front of me, I felt like jumping from one piece of ice to another piece of ice.

Discovering curiosity about how I resist as a White, professional person to seek out information about racism, instead I expect the Black presenter to give it to me. Recognizing I am entitled to be "taken care of" when learning about race.

As the Black client in both demonstration role-plays, I had my strongest reactions to the Compliant Leader. I discovered how patronized and infantilized I felt by the compliant White clinician and found myself turning to the audience, stepping out of my role in the role-play, to express my dissatisfaction and annoyance, saying "See what I have to put up with!"

In the last ten minutes of SLSDD, a White woman (R) voiced how angry she was about our asking them to do the exercise. A White male quickly added that he had refused to participate. After the workshop, R reported having felt sick in her body when she did the role-play. It was clear the sick feeling was a reaction to feeling the dominant or compliant role. Thinking isomorphy, both voices were quite important in helping us see how challenging it is when we let ourselves see and feel the impact of how we easily maintain the power hierarchies that enact and continue racist norms. These voices surfaced the subgroup voice in many of us of the challenge of seeing and feeling our part in maintaining racism in everyday life or even more importantly in therapeutic interactions. It is this level of emotional experience that SCT sees as imperative in training group leaders as otherwise we will continue to perpetuate the cultural norms that maintain racism by enacting our closed survivor-roles related to power and control.

Lastly, in this same training, we recognized afterwards the isomorphic racialized survivor-roles that were enacted in the workshop itself: our leadership system outputs induced care-taking roles toward the Black female leader and anger and scapegoating toward the White leaders. None of this was planned, yet inevitably as SCT emphasizes, we enact the dynamics that we do not explore. Not surprisingly since we were focused on the authority phase survivor-roles that enact racism, these same survivor-roles emerged in relationship to us as leaders, usefully moving beyond role-playing to life. One participant voiced both wanting the black female leader who presented anti-racist material to care-take the group by giving the group "more" and wanting to get rid of the White leaders who were introducing a difficult exercise. This was a useful learning for us to see the isomorphy even though we only understood it afterwards as a racialized splitting and elicitation of care-taking.

All three of these "workshops" have helped us in different ways to understand the importance and the ongoing challenges of training group leaders in working with survivor-roles with an awareness of their racialized dimensions and implicit goals of maintaining what is, i.e., racism.

Intersectionality

Looking at intersectionality as formulated by Crenshaw et al. (1995) through TLHS, we have drawn from Gaun et al. (2021): "Intersectionality is a theoretical framework that investigates how interlocking systems of power and oppression at the societal level influence the lived experiences of historically and socially marginalized groups" (p. 1). Exploring authority phase group dynamics inevitably reflects the interlocking dynamics of power, control, and oppression at the societal level, and again at the level internalized by survivor-roles in each person.[12] Intersectionality is imperative for leaders and members as part of recognizing the context of individual survivor-roles and their origin. SCT works with the complexities of the role origins in the work phase, building on the resources the group has developed in the authority and intimacy phases. In the work phase, group members explore seeing themselves in the context of their history.

Ethical Considerations

Though psychology has been slow to work with the ethical/clinical issues of racism in psychotherapy (Drustrup, 2020), focus on anti-racism as essential for ethical practice (Ribeiro, 2021) is increasing. Social workers are trained in anti-racist practices and in exploring internalized racial biases and manifestations, yet often from an "individual ethnic or cultural identity and lack conceptual, historical, and sociological knowledge about racism" (Varghese, 2016, p. S134). Exploration of ethical issues around racism for practitioners who train group leaders in experiential group training is essential.

In training group leaders, SCT emphasizes the importance of legitimizing, humanizing, de-pathologizing, contextualizing, and normalizing all human experience, all of which help create an exploratory context in which racism can be acknowledged and explored. SCT leaders learn to develop collaborative systems with their groups, providing an antidote to colonialized, dominant leadership. This is not easy, as all leaders and group members have developed closed survivor-roles in our context of racialized power dynamics. In addition, SCT leaders introduce methods and structures that when not introduced collaboratively or in misattunement can easily be misapplied from closed-survivor roles that enact the power dynamics that underlie racism and other forms of oppression. SCT's four basic methods (contextualizing, FSG, boundarying, vectoring), when introduced in attunement to the group and its members, are all useful in building an ethical, humanizing group context for exploring racism and the closed survivor-roles which maintain colonizing patterns.

Implications for Training

Establishing group norms that support curiosity about our closed survivor-roles fosters exploration about how we, often unknowingly, keep cultural/racist structures and function intact. Racism and colonizing norms imprison all living human systems in survival, maintaining what is. Building on Stoute (2022), enacting [through what SCT calls survivor-roles] that devalues Blackness maintains our [communal racialized trauma] "with sadistic domination of the racialized other." Without developing our groups so that we can explore our sadism and masochism, and our dominant or compliant roles, we will continue to enact them and remain complicit with the racist norms implicit in our closed survivor-roles in the authority phase. By failing to recognize and explore how our closed survivor-roles are triggered by group dynamics and also maintain the very group dynamics that enact racism and sadism, we continue to perpetuate what is.

Education in racism matters, yet it is far from enough to change the enactment of everyday racist norms. Instead, experiential training of group therapists is essential for changing system norms, up and down the hierarchy of living human systems. In training group leaders, how do we activate curiosity about racism and how it emerges in the everyday life of our groups? Only from a curious place can our boundaries open so that we can explore, rather than prohibit the closed survivor-roles we have all developed in our racist cultures. Only through exploring these roles can we develop these roles and weaken the repetition compulsions that the closed roles maintain. Closed survivor-roles are our psychological/ neurobiological adaptations to our context: they live in our bodies, filter how we see the world, how we relate with others and to ourselves, and when we open our boundaries and when we close them.

Unlike Stoute (2022) and Paul (1996), who describe how hate is metabolized through the prohibitions of super ego, SCT works with the *exploration* of hate in the crisis of hatred with the leader, as an alternative pathway for metabolizing hatred that leads to creativity and fellowship (de Maré et al., 1991), making it less likely that we will transfer destructive hate trans-generationally. When training groups fail to develop the capacity to explore and metabolize sadism and hatred, the dominance hierarchies established by Europeans, enacted in the slave trade and in the colonization of the United States and still actively enacted in many current U.S. systems, will continue to be maintained. As Paul (1996) notes, when hate is not metabolized, lynching is implicitly sanctioned.

It is in the group process where we can discover the racial enactments we had "forgotten," as Stoute (2022) terms it, by remembering in the "transference through action" and not words as we are "all deconditioned to racial violence . . . [and do] not recognize the sadism of everyday cultural enactments."

Working with the here-and-now expression of our survivor-roles, SCT is exploring how our culture's racist structures emerge in group dynamics and are maintained by these same dynamics in a recapitulation of our closed survivor-roles. Drawing from Stoute (2022, 2023), enacting roles that devalue Blackness maintains our communal racialized trauma with sadistic domination of the "racialized other." We would add, by exploring these roles, we can develop our survivor-roles and influence our groups functioning in the direction of anti-racism.

For example, noticing when our boundaries have closed, do we get critical of ourselves? Self-criticism without seeing the context is self-centered. Or do we get critical and blame others without seeing the context? Or do we access curiosity about how the larger system context and its norms are impacting all of us and how our survivor-roles are perpetuating the context and its implicit and explicit racism?

Next Steps for Us All

As group therapists, we have a unique context for understanding how group dynamics enact and maintain racism. An essential next step is to see how to use what we know in the service of weakening racism and developing decolonizing groups.

We end with a quote from a participant's reflections about her experience in our most recent workshop. It captures intersectionality and the heart of our challenge as group leaders and trainers to move beyond education alone and the implicit racism of "trying to get it right" and instead build groups in which we can work with racism as it emerges in ourselves and our groups, knowing that it will. By developing groups that learn from this emergence and move from surviving, to developing and transforming our survivor-roles, we move closer to transforming the racist systems in which we all participate:

This whitewater ride—from a huge anger to a teary collapse—in the face of the over-whelmingly powerful Other—is an awfully familiar route. I have known this, not just between Blacks and Whites in the US, but between Russians and Koreans in the former USSR, and in Putin's Russia of today.[13] I have travelled down this wretched path more times than I can count (though in all truth, I never did count; the beauty of complete collapse is that it wipes all memory clean). But now I remember. And now I see that there exists one crucial difference: this time, in this exercise with two White men, I was *not alone* in my attempt to retrace and understand the journey.

And with this realization, I am IN! No longer a mere onlooker, a smug judge, or a guilty bystander, I am ALL in. *Let's do it! Let's at least try to do it in a way that writes a different ending to the story.*

Will we be able to get it right the next time around? And then, a realization, painful and joyous in equal parts: *No, we will not* get it right. Again and again, we will get it wrong—and *that is a source of our hope!* Because working with and weakening racialized role-locks can only be done in the present, when we catch ourselves doing the very thing we set out to undo. Because the only dynamics of race we can change are the ones that we still carry in our bodies and continue to enact in our relationships. Because, regardless of what we *say* racism is, the ruptures and genuine repairs of connection are the only places where we can truly know and slowly un-learn its painful truth (Shulgina, 2023).

Endnotes

1 A theory of living human systems can be applied to any living human system as small as a single person or as large as a country or even the world-as-a-whole.
2 We substitute the word "identifying" for "discriminating" given the latter's meaning in racialized contexts.
3 In SCT, projections are outputs from a closed-survivor role.

4   Once cognitive defenses are undone, SCT groups work with the somatic defenses, starting first with tension.

5   Somatic and dissociative defenses common in racialized trauma are also worked with in this phase.

6   Exploring hatred and sadism frees the group from the survivor-roles which have defended against this experience and when explored in FSG, the group and its members develop much greater capacity to know their sadism rather than defending against it in repression or acting it out.

7   Our emphasis on the group dynamics maintaining racism was echoed by a recent article in the NY Times: When Congress was discussing emancipating slaves, an objection was raised "warning that 'the next step would be to raise the Negroes to a social and political equality with whites; and [if done] . . . we would soon find the present condition of the two races reversed.' Black Americans would be masters and white people slaves." (Kennedy, 2023). [We would note that the dynamic belief here implies colonization as the inevitable norm.]

8   In this workshop, all participants had some basic knowledge of SCT. We have not yet introduced this to those without prior experience in SCT and would not recommend doing so as having the basics of SCT builds the resources for this more complex application of the protocol.

9   Attendees in this workshop were predominantly White.

10   SCT uses the structure of SLSDD at the end of all group sessions to contain the work and shift from exploring to observing and integrating.

11   SCT (Agazarian, 1997) introduces a set of questions that enable people to learn to undo their anxiety, beginning by asking about the source of the anxiety: is your anxiety coming from something you are thinking, a feeling or sensation in your body, or being at the edge of the unknown where we all get anxious? Paradoxically, the intent of the anxiety protocol is to empower the client by giving them a skill to use with themselves yet the racist role enactments use the protocol in the service of domination.

12   It is common that in each subphase, e.g., flight or fight, members identify different survivor roles.

13   In Russia, the history of the Korean community is scarred by Stalin's perception of the "Asian threat to Soviet security," targeted ethnic cleansings, forced relocation, exclusion from military service, and access only to the humanities branches of university learning. While legal restrictions to Korean rights in Russia were lifted during 1953–1975, the implicit prohibition of professional advancement, racial discrimination, and political oppression have continued well into the present. The law about rehabilitation of the victims of political repression in Russia was issued in 1991. It was applied to Koreans in 1993. My family received its Certificate of Rehabilitation in 2018.

References

Adams, J. M., Carter, F. B., & Gantt, S. P. (2023, March 25–31). *Whatever we say a thing isn't, it IS! (Adapted from Korzybski, 1933): Weakening racialized role locks in SCT practice.* [Conference workshop.] SCT Annual Conference, Philadelphia, PA. www.systemscentered.com/SCT-Conference-2023/Program-Workshops.

Agazarian, Y. M. (1997). *Systems-centered therapy for groups.* New York: Guilford. Re-printed in paperback (2004). London: Karnac Books.

Agazarian, Y. M. & Gantt, S. P. (2003). Phases of group development: Systems-centered hypotheses and their implications for research and practice. *Group Dynamics: Theory, Research and Practice, 7*(3), 238–252. https://doi.org/10.1037/1089-2699.7.3.238.

Agazarian, Y. M., Gantt, S. P., & Carter, F. B. (2021). *Systems-centered training: An illustrated guide for applying a theory of living human systems.* London, UK: Routledge.

Ashley, W. W. C. (2021). *New rules for radicals: TNT for faith-based leaders.* King of Prussia, PA: Judson Press.

Ashley, W. W. C., Gantt, S. P., Adams, J. M., & Carter, F. B. (2022, April 2–8). *Working with systemic racism and its impact* [Conference workshop]. SCT Annual Conference, online. www.systemscentered.com/SCT-Conference-2022/2022-Program-Workshops.

Crenshaw, K., Gotanda, N., Peller, G., & Thomas, K. (Eds). (1995). *Critical race theory: The key writings that formed the movement.* The New Press.

De Maré, P., Piper, R., & Thompson, S. (1991). *Koinonia: From hate, through dialogue, to culture in the large group.* Karnac Books.

Drustrup, D. (2020). White therapists addressing racism in psychotherapy: An ethical and clinical model for practice. *Ethics & Behavior, 30*(3), 181–196. https://doi.org/10.1080/10508422.2019.1588732.

EmbraceRace. (2020, May 30). *This graphic is adapted by Ellen Tuzzolo from an original graphic published by the Safehouse Progressive Alliance for Nonviolence* [Infographic]. Facebook. www.facebook.com/photo/?fbid=3307589285932578&set=this-graphic-is-adapted-by-ellen-tuzzolo-from-an-original-graphic-published-by-t

Finlay, L. D., Abernethy, A. D., & Garrels, S. R. (2016). Scapegoating in group therapy: Insights from Girard's mimetic theory. *International Journal of Group Psychotherapy, 66*(2), 188–204. https://doi.org/10.1080/00207284.2015.1106174.

Flores, P. J. (2010). Group psychotherapy and neuro-plasticity: An attachment theory perspective. *International Journal of Group Psychotherapy, 60*(4), 546–570. https://doi.org/10.1521/ijgp.2010.60.4.546.

Gantt, S. P. (2018). Developing groups that change our minds and transform our brains: Systems-centered's functional subgrouping, its impact on our neurobiology, and its role in each phase of group development. *Psychoanalytic Inquiry: Today's Bridge Between Psychoanalysis and the Group World [Special Issue], 38*(4), 270–284. https://doi.org/10.1080/07351690.2018.1444851.

Gantt, S. P. (2019). Implications of neuroscience for group psychotherapy. In F. J. Kaklauskas & L.R. Greene (Eds), *Core principles of group psychotherapy: An integrated theory, research, and practice training manual* (pp. 156–170). New York: Routledge.

Gantt, S. P. (2021). Systems-centered theory (SCT) into group therapy: Beyond surviving ruptures to repairing and thriving. *International Journal of Group Psychotherapy, 71*(2), 224–252. https://doi.org/10.1080/00207284.2020.1772073.

Gantt, S. P. & Adams, J. M. (2010). Systems-centered training for therapists: Beyond stereotyping to integrating diversities into the change process. *Women & Therapy, 33*(1), 101–120. https://doi.org/10.1080/02703140903404812.

Gantt, S. P. & Agazarian, Y. M. (2010). Developing the group mind through functional subgrouping: Linking systems-centered training (SCT) and interpersonal neurobiology. *International Journal of Group Psychotherapy, 60*(4), 515–544. https://doi.org/10.1521/ijgp.2010.60.4.515.

Gantt, S. P., Carter, F. B., Gibbons, D., & Hartford, R. (2021, October 24). *Systems-centered training & therapy: Seeing the system, not just people. Commemorating the work of Yvonne Agazarian.* [Online event.] Systems-Centered Training & Research Institute. www.systemscentered.com/Training/View-Single-Event/ID/5595.

Gaun, A., Thomas, M., Vittinghoff, E., Bowleg, L., Mangurian, C., & Wesson, P. (2021). An investigation of quantitative methods for assessing intersectionality in health research: A systematic review. *SSM-Population Health, 16.* https://doi.org/10.1016/j.ssmph.2021.100977.

Kennedy, R. (2023, June 7). The truth is, many Americans just don't want Black people to get ahead. *The New York Times.* www.nytimes.com/2023/06/07/opinion/resistance-black-advancement-affirmative-action.html.

Major, B. & Barndt, J. (2023). *Deconstructing racism: A path toward lasting change.* Minneapolis, MN: Fortress Press.

Menakem, R. (2017). *My grandmother's hands: Racialized trauma and the pathway to mending our hearts and bodies.* Las Vegas, NV: Central Recovery Press.

Paul, R. A. (1996). *Moses and civilization: The meaning behind Freud's myth.* New Haven, CT: Yale University Press.

Ribeiro, M. D. (2021). Intentional call to action: Mindfully discussing race in group psychotherapy. *The American Journal of Psychotherapy, 74*(2), 89–96. https://doi.org/10.1176/appi.psychotherapy.20200041.

Shulgina, N. A. (2023). Whatever we say a thing is . . . may not matter as much as we think it does: An uncensored response to the last 2023 SCT conference workshop. *Systems-Centered News, 31*(2), 17–20.

Stoute, B. J. (2022, October 9). *Black rage, out rage: Mitigating the colonial mindset.* [Online event]. Freud Museum World Mental Health Day 2022. www.freud.org.uk/event/refugees-primitiveness-and-the-eurocentric-gaze.

Stoute, B. J. (2023). How our mind becomes racialized: Implications for the therapeutic encounter. In H. Crisp & G. O. Gabbard (Eds), *Gabbard's textbook of psychotherapeutic treatments* (2nd Edition., pp. 575–605). Washington, D.C.: American Psychiatric Association Publishing.

Varghese, R. (2016). Teaching to transform? Addressing race and racism in the teaching of clinical social work practice. *Journal of Social Work Education, 52*(sup1), S134–S147. https://doi.org/10.10 80/10437797.2016.1174646.

Acknowledgements

Figures 2.1–2.5 are copyrighted by the Systems-Centered Training and Research Institute (SCTRI) and reprinted here with permission of SCTRI.

Figure 2.6 is copyrighted by Susan P. Gantt and reprinted here with her permission.

SCT® and Systems-Centered® are registered trademarks of the Systems-Centered Training and Research Institute, Inc., a non-profit organization.

Much appreciation to Kathy Lum for her tireless work in supporting us bringing this chapter to life and to Miles Agag for his skill in translating our ideas for illustrations into real illustrations.

3 Adopting a Multicultural Orientation to Work with International Students of Color in Heterogeneous Interpersonal Process Groups

Kristin M. Miserocchi and Yujia Lei

Cultural Heterogeneity of International Students of Color

International students of Color (ISC) comprise more than 70 percent of the total international student population in the U.S. (National Association of Foreign Student Advisers, 2020), with over half coming from countries in Asia (Open Doors, 2022). For the purposes of this chapter, we define ISC as undergraduate and graduate students of Color in the U.S. on a non-immigrant visa. Historically, international students are inappropriately treated as a homogeneous group, which effectively erases their breadth of diversity, such as language, religious and spiritual beliefs, cultural values, communication styles, and socioeconomic status. In addition, reducing these groups to "whole-race" categories (e.g., Black, Asian, White, Latinx/Hispanic) erases regional diversity, dimensions of identity, and privilege-based hierarchies within larger racial and ethnic groups (Blum, 2015, p. 87).

ISC get little credit for all they contribute to U.S. higher educational institutions, and to U.S. society as a whole. They increase diversity of thought and perspective, contribute intellectually, have a significant impact on the U.S. economy, and ". . . ultimately benefit the good will between countries" (Lee & Rice, 2007, p. 381; Yang, 2020). However, research has found some predictable patterns of stress that tend to emerge for many international students, centered on adjustment and belonging. Leaving what is familiar and being immersed in the unfamiliar can trigger a wide range of adjustment concerns, such as language proficiency, limited diet/nutrition options, navigation of new physical spaces (e.g., university campus, a new city, public transportation), adapting to a new educational system (e.g., emphasis on critical thinking and class participation, different teaching methods and grading system), and living self-sufficiently for the first time (Walker & Conyne, 2007; Yakunina, et al., 2011). Moving away from one's home community to a new community can trigger a sense of isolation and loneliness, especially if members of that new community misunderstand or prejudge the international heritage of international students. These adjustments and belonging issues can have a significant impact on their day-to-day lives, academic and interpersonal functioning, as well as holistic well-being.

Intersectionality—Country of Origin and Race/Ethnicity

According to Yao and colleagues (2018), "International students to the U.S., particularly those from non-White and non-English speaking countries, are often othered and racialized using U.S. constructs of race" (p. 39). This reflects a global racial hierarchy that privileges Anglo-Saxon and European identities and denigrates BIPOC (Black, Indigenous, People of Color) identities (Glass et al., 2022; Lee & Rice, 2007; Yao et al., 2018). Lee and Rice (2007) explore this dynamic through the lens of neo-racism, which combines phenotypic-based

DOI: 10.4324/9781003455783-5

racism (i.e., based on physical or observable traits) with xenophobic and nativist prejudice and discrimination. Thus, study abroad experiences for international students vary based on phenotypic characteristics (e.g., skin color, hair), country of origin, religious and cultural practices, and the political relationship between their home and host countries.

Uprooting one's life, moving away from familiar communities, and immersing oneself in a foreign land would be stressful for just about anybody; however, having to navigate neo-racism exacerbates an already stressful situation for ISC (Lee & Rice, 2007; Yao et al., 2018). Research has found that these students experience covert and overt forms of prejudice and discrimination, including insults, disrespectful treatment, a lack of formal and informal support, assumptions about their competence, and stereotypes and micro-aggressions (Lee & Rice, 2007; Yao et al., 2018). Additionally, for many ISC, this is their first time experiencing the stress and marginalization that comes with being a Person of Color in the U.S. (Lee & Rice, 2007; Yao et al., 2018; Yeo et al., 2019). This can feel like a significant shock to the system since they lack the emotional and psychological calluses of their BIPOC domestic student counterparts, who have been socialized in a White supremacist society their entire lives. ISC coming to university counseling centers for support may not have the words or awareness to describe this insidious neo-racist dynamic. Instead, these students may present symptoms that simply look like depression, anxiety, social anxiety, and adjustment, etc. Therefore, the responsibility lies on the shoulders of the therapist to take neo-racism into consideration when conceptualizing these symptoms to avoid engaging in treatment that is disaffirming, exclusive, and reinforcing of neo-racist narratives about ISC.

Given the hostility these students encounter on a regular basis, putting the responsibility on the shoulders of ISC to adapt is absurd and cruel, and yet, this is exactly what is often expected by their higher educational institutions and recommended in the literature (George Mwangi & English, 2017; Lee & Rice, 2007; Yao et al., 2018). ISC are expected to find ways to assimilate as a way of coping with or reducing acculturation stress, even though individual and systemic-level neo-racism make complete assimilation impossible for these students. While research has found it beneficial for international students to engage in both acculturation and enculturation processes (i.e., connecting with aspects of both the new and home cultures), this type of integration is ultimately limited if ". . . the environment is not conducive to developing bicultural competency" (Yoon et al., 2013, p. 28).

Members from a culturally diverse group will notice visible differences (e.g., skin color, accent, non-verbal language) from the start of group therapy, and will attune to cues alluding to invisible differences (e.g., country of origin, religion and spirituality, sexuality). For example, Serena, an African American female, said to Bernard that she was glad to see other Black people in the group. Group therapists observed that Bernard was not as excited and seemed hesitant to say something. With facilitation, Bernard shared that he was an international student and his family immigrated to Canada from Haiti when he was ten. With no discernible accent like many international students, he reported that he often chooses to "pass" as African American in many social situations, despite his desire to be accepted for who he is. This led to a conversation about their different definitions and experiences of being Black, and the impact of racism and neo-racism on their mental health.

International Students and Group Therapy

As mentioned, many international students suffer significant stress stemming from a lack of belonging. Unfortunately, research suggests that international students are underutilizing formal systems of support, like mental health services (Walker & Conyne, 2007; Yakunina et al., 2011). International students who engage in mental health services, specifically group therapy, experience a wealth of benefits, such as affirmation of their lived experience, connection with others, interpersonal learning and skill-building, increased self-awareness, and social support and resources. Researchers have found great value in support groups, as well as psychoeducational/skills groups (Delgado-Romero & Wu, 2010; Walker & Conyne, 2007; Yakunina et al., 2011; Yau, 2004). Some of the benefits these types of groups offer include: opportunities to feel validated and less alone; education about U.S. culture; and adaptive coping strategies to assist with assimilation (e.g., cross-cultural communication, adjustment, assertive training, dating).

Although we agree with the research that these types of groups are beneficial for international students, we want to emphasize the benefits of interpersonal process (IP) groups. In contrast to psychoeducational/skills groups, IP groups offer an unstructured group experience focused on here-and-now group dynamics. This type of group format creates space for ISC to share their life narratives, examine interpersonal related concerns, and give/receive interpersonal feedback. Another benefit is the interpersonal focus of these groups, centering the importance of the relationship dynamics amongst group members and leaders. This relationship focus aligns well with a more collectivistic orientation present in many of the countries that are home to ISC (Bemak & Chung, 2015). Thus, we believe that IP groups have the potential to offer ISC a more individual and personalized experience, suitable for such a diverse and heterogeneous group (Ribeiro, 2020).

Conceptual Framework

We will reference and integrate the multicultural orientation (MCO) framework to help us conceptualize our clinical examples. MCO is a therapist's attunement to relevant cultural issues and dynamics in session, described as a "way of being" with clients (Owen et al., 2011, p. 274). Rather than guided by a therapist's skill level and knowledge (i.e., multicultural competence), MCO touches on the therapist's belief that culture is always salient in therapy and deserving of attention. This idea is also emphasized by the Association for Specialists in Group Work (ASGW), stating that group therapists are responsible for ". . . the ongoing task of acknowledging that dynamics of both culture and power are inherent in any group setting" (Guth et al., 2019, p. 8).

The MCO framework is broken down into three interrelated components: cultural humility, cultural comfort, and cultural opportunities. Cultural humility involves ". . . openness, self-awareness, being egoless, and incorporating self-reflection and critique after willingly interacting with diverse individuals" (Foronda et al., 2016, p. 213). Being both other-oriented (i.e., curious and open) and self-reflective (i.e., critiquing and humble) serve to dismantle power dynamics that can interfere with the cultivation of the therapist-client partnership (Foronda et al., 2016). Mosher and colleagues (2017) suggest that the first step toward cultural humility is for therapists to engage in critical self-examination and self-awareness to facilitate a deeper understanding of how their own cultural experiences impact their view of self, others, and the world. Cultural humility has proved a positive force in strengthening the therapeutic relationship through the therapist's willingness to prioritize culture and learn from the client (Davis et al., 2018; Hook, et al., 2013; Mosher et al., 2017). Additionally, cultural humility can facilitate repair of cultural-based ruptures in the context of the therapeutic relationship. A culturally humble therapist rejects the expert role and embraces transparency and openness, a dynamic that lays the foundation for clients to give corrective/

suggestive feedback to the therapist (Mosher et al., 2017). Finally, a cultural humility orientation helps therapists navigate cultural differences that could potentially lead to tension or conflict (Mosher et al., 2017). Adopting an other-orientation necessarily means that the therapists prioritize understanding the client's cultural worldview over imposing their own cultural worldview, even if those values seem to be in conflict.

The remaining two components of the MCO framework are what Davis and colleagues (2018) describe as the "behavioral expressions of cultural humility" (p. 92). **Cultural comfort** refers to a therapist's ease and openness in situations where culture is salient and is a natural outcome of orienting toward cultural humility (Davis et al., 2018). These authors add that the presence of discomfort in these types of situations can alert the therapist to potential growth opportunities. **Cultural opportunities** are ever-present opportunities to explore and attend to clients' important cultural identities in session (Davis et al., 2018). While these can be either client or therapist-initiated conversations, research suggests that clients have better outcomes when their therapists seize upon opportunities to initiate conversations or further explore cultural issues with their clients (Owen et al., 2016).

Group Interventions

Adopting the MCO Framework for Group Therapy with ISC

Now that we understand the MCO framework on a conceptual basis, the next step is to understand how the three pillars of this framework (cultural humility, cultural comfort, and cultural opportunities) are linked with group interventions and dynamics. Members who perceive group therapy as a place where they cannot freely express their cultural identities will likely find it less beneficial. This implies that implementing interventions in group therapy aimed at encouraging clients from diverse cultural backgrounds to authentically express themselves can enhance the effectiveness of group therapy (Rigg & Kivlighan, 2022).

Group therapists should be willing to engage flexibly and intentionally with ISC. Although this chapter focuses on ISC as group members, ISC may be group therapists as well and in addition to ISC spaces, ISC colleagues offer invaluable insights (Yakunina et al., 2011; Yau, 2004). Meeting ISC where they are offers group therapists the opportunity to identify potential benefits of group therapy from their perspective and instill hope, which could increase buy-in. Group therapists may also need to adapt informed consent procedures in order to talk extensively with potential members about what to expect out of the group therapy experience (including confidentiality and privacy; Yakunina et al., 2011; Yau, 2004).

Group therapists need to be vigilant to avoid stereotyping, over-generalizing, and over-pathologizing ISC, and they need to be attuned to instances when group members may be doing the same thing. Additionally, group therapists need to be cautious about over-focusing on coping strategies to manage acculturation stress or expecting ISC to change or assimilate. As discussed, if ISC do not feel the group therapy space is safe and inclusive, they will not open up (i.e., they will engage in cultural concealment), and will not benefit from the group to the fullest extent possible (Kivlighan et al., 2019b). Chen and Rybak (2018) talk about the importance of group therapists fluidly shifting in and out of the observer/facilitator and participant roles, which applies here. Sometimes group therapists will need to illuminate group processes occurring here-and-now, and sometimes they will need to self-disclose their reactions, just as they expect of group members. Always staying grounded in an other-orientation will ensure group therapists are operating with openness and curiosity, as opposed to expertise and knowledge that is characteristic of a "colonial imperialist mentality" and can thrust the group leaders into an oppressive role (Bemak and Chung, 2015, p. 12).

MCO Framework Applied to Group Therapy Development and Dynamics

In the following section, we will discuss how the MCO framework can be integrated with group interventions throughout the developmental stages of a group, first identified by Tuckman (1965) and further delineated by Chen and Rybak (2018). We will highlight how to integrate the MCO framework into: 1) the forming stage via group preparation, introductions, and norming processes; 2) the storming stage with a discussion of interventions aimed at navigating and conflict; 3) the norming stage via interventions that cultivate safety and group cohesion; and 4) the performing stage by highlighting interventions focused on interpersonal learning and healing. We will center considerations for ISC in these group spaces, though we believe adopting the MCO framework gives therapists the flexibility and capabilities to work with anyone in any type of group.

Forming Stage: Group Preparation and Orientation

The tasks in this stage of the group involve orientation, establishing norms, getting to know one another, and beginning to cultivate safety and connection (Chen & Rybak, 2018; Tuckman, 1965). A sense of universality will likely emerge right away, challenging group members' beliefs that they are unique in their suffering (Yalom & Leszcz, 2020). One of the earliest ways to shine the spotlight on culture is through the norming process, both in the pre-group meeting and in the first group session. This process serves to orient members to the culture and expectations of group therapy. In the pre-group meeting, group therapists can invite ISC to share about themselves as cultural beings, as well as any concerns these potential members may have going into groups. For instance, in our pre-group meeting with Haru, an international graduate student from Japan, he expressed worry about his ability to communicate effectively and understand others speaking English. As a result, he explained, many perceived him as introverted and shy. We validated his concerns and attempted to reassure him by talking about diversity present in the group and the wide range of non-verbal ways to communicate. We also discussed the group as a laboratory for him to practice both English-speaking and his assertiveness skills to meet his needs (e.g., asking for members to repeat themselves, sharing his lived experience, receiving feedback on his communication effectiveness). The MCO framework gives group therapists the tools they need to be more attuned to the culturally relevant dynamics present for each member and for the group as a whole. Group therapists' willingness to center culture right away is a demonstration of all three components of the MCO framework, and is in alignment with the strategies set forth by the ASGW (Guth et al., 2019). This not only grounds the potential group member in the expectations and norms of the group, but it also begins the work of increasing their own cultural comfort.

Spotlighting cultural relevance can be put into practice right away in the first session, as a part of introductions. To make these introductions culturally relevant and meaningful, both group members and therapists can share any salient identities that they want the others to know. Group therapists can also invite members to share their observations about the diversity of the group, and encourage them to express curiosity about one another by asking open questions. Setting up introductions in this way will allow group therapists and members to engage in self-reflection on their own salient identities, avoid making assumptions about others' identities, and interact with curiosity and openness, all aspects of cultural humility. This type of introduction also has the benefit of continuing to cultivate cultural comfort, on the part of the group therapists and members, as well as potentially opening up cultural opportunities for further and more in-depth discussions.

Group therapists can formalize cultural humility as a norm by including it on paperwork distributed to group members (e.g., group agreements or contracts, educational handouts). Also, group therapists can offer a definition and work collaboratively with members to operationalize cultural humility in the group space. This conversation can help group members gain insight into their own internal cues, as well as observable verbal and non-verbal cues, to gauge the presence or absence of cultural humility and comfort. This norming process is illustrated in the following brief example from the first session of a heterogeneous IP group. Fatima talked about coming from Saudi Arabia and wearing a hijab, despite now exploring her feminist identity and religious beliefs. She talked about her fear of being judged by her family, and feelings of loneliness from her lack of in-depth connections with her American cohort. She also talked about feeling pressured to represent the entire Muslim community. Group therapists expressed appreciation for Fatima's disclosure and invited all group members to share their own worries about being prejudged based on cultural factors, both in and out of the group.

As a fruitful conclusion to this conversation, group therapists and members collaborated to add the "Cultural Relevance" to the current group norms. Together we broke down what cultural relevance might look like in our group space: 1) Speaking only from one's own experience, with no self or other-imposed pressure to justify, defend, or represent one's background, heritage, or culture; 2) seeing each other as fully intersectional, with all identities welcomed into the space; and 3) keeping the group space rooted in subjective personal experiences, to avoid a discussion turning into a political debate. This discussion around "Cultural Relevance" has been a launching pad for the authors to more intentionally foster cultural humility as a norm in subsequent group therapy experiences. In the early stages of group, group leaders need to be more directive to help increase mutual engagement and facilitate early bonding, and increase group awareness and intentionality around culturally humble ways of interacting (Chen & Rybak, 2018). This might include effective prompts, shifting to a group focus, inviting participation from others, and highlighting non-verbals. For example, to foster curiosity among members, leaders might gently invite and remind members to check in with each other (with consent), e.g., "I wonder if you'd like to ask Andy a question, Claire?" To help members adopt an other-orientation, group leaders could invite members to use mentalization, particularly the White domestic group members, e.g. "What do you imagine Adisa feels being one of the only international students from Nigeria on-campus?" Like cultural humility, mentalization is both self and other focused, relies on openness and curiosity, and is oriented in the here-and-now (Bateman et al., 2018). According to Grimes and Kivlighan (2022), it is not enough for cultural humility to only be adopted by the group therapists, it must also be adopted as a guiding principle of the group as a whole.

Storming Stage: Navigating Tension/Conflict and Leaning into Difference

Encountering something different, unexpected, or unfamiliar can be a triggering experience for people. As the novelty of universality and validation wears off, tension will start to become apparent in this stage as members become aware of perceived differences, potentially leading to projection and conflict (Chen & Rybak, 2018; Yalom & Leszcz, 2020).

While successfully navigating tension and conflict is helpful for interpersonal learning and healing, it also means problematic ways of interacting with others will be reenacted in the group. In the absence of cultural humility and without therapist intervention, this reenactment will become harmful to members from marginalized backgrounds and will interfere with the cultivation of deep bonds (Guth et al., 2019; PettyJohn et al., 2020). The absence of cultural humility can reinforce the invisible White supremacy in the IP groups, which could have a significant negative impact on ISC by contributing to unaddressed microaggressions, isolation and alienation, cultural assimilation pressure, stereotyping, and making assumptions. According to PettyJohn and colleagues, ". . . therapists who avoid or do not bring up notable differences in privilege may inadvertently come off as more authoritarian, unresponsive, unwilling to listen, or untrustworthy . . ." (p. 317). In this type of group environment, we believe that group members occupying marginalized identities will also see more privileged group members in similar ways—authoritarian, unresponsive, unwilling to listen, and untrustworthy. A potential source of harm is feeling othered, which is an emotional and psychological wound overemphasizing ways we are different (Logan, 2020). Othering is perpetuated when we pull away from others in reaction to difference, as opposed to leaning into difference with curiosity. For instance, consider an IP group composed of almost all White, domestic students and one ISC. Based on our previous discussion, this international student likely already feels a sense of otherness and alienation in their day-to-day life. If not addressed, the therapist and privileged group members are at risk of reenacting this student's daily lived experience in the group—an experience that would only serve to reinforce that student's burgeoning belief that they truly are an outsider.

The group at this stage is also vulnerable to cultural misinterpretations and misunderstandings, which can occur when privileged members assume all members share their values and socialization (Chen & Rybak, 2018). This might look like differences in: rate of speech, level of directness or bluntness, emotional expressions, comfort with vulnerability or openness, or individualistic vs collectivist ways of interacting with the world at large. For instance, an ISC who is more reserved or quiet might elicit in other members insecurities ("Am I talking too much?") or suspicion ("Are they trustworthy?"). If members entertain these fears, rather than expressing curiosity about the quiet member, they might potentially draw inaccurate conclusions and miss an opportunity, in this case, to learn that the quiet member was engaging his/her active listening skills and staying quiet as a sign of respect. Without intervention from the group therapists, the ripple effects from an interaction like this could significantly impair the ability of the group to bond and become cohesive.

Tension and conflict in group spaces are inevitable and, if handled properly, also a catalyst for change and growth (Brabender & MacNair-Semands, 2022; Chen & Rybak, 2018; Yalom & Leszcz, 2020). Yalom and Leszcz state, "The therapist's task is to harness conflict and use it in the service of growth" (p. 449). Effectively navigating tension and conflict, requires group therapists to pay attention and illuminate the process; co-regulate their emotional reactions along with the group members; validate and invite the sharing of reactions; and apply here-and-now learning to members' lives outside of group (Chen & Rybak, 2018). Research has found that engaging humbly with someone enhances conflict resolution and increases the likelihood of forgiveness (Davis et al., 2013). Thus, orienting toward the already established cultural humility norm can help navigate these choppy waters when culture is relevant to the tension or conflict. With this approach, curiosity, understanding, and reconciliation become the goals of the interaction, rather than defending oneself or changing another's opinion. Slowing down the members' urge to react and get them to orient to each other will facilitate active listening, increase the likelihood for greater understanding, open up opportunities to give and receive empathy, and help members transcend cultural differences.

Norming Stage: Cultivating a Safe and Cohesive Space

As the group matures, members will become less reactive to perceived differences and more interested and curious about one another. IP groups offer opportunities to practice seeing others as part of an us/we instead of a them/other. Chen and Rybak (2018) describe group cohesiveness as the sense of "we" in the group, in other words the strong bonds that unite all individual members together as a whole. Attuning to cultural factors, building emotional intimacy, and engaging in self-disclosure all positively contribute to the cohesiveness and safety of the group, which, in turn, improves therapy outcomes (Yalom & Leszcz, 2020). The cohesion and safety of the group stem from a self-reinforcing trust cycle: "trust → self-disclosure → empathy → acceptance → trust" (Yalom & Leszcz, 2020, p. 77). Member self-disclosure is a necessary mechanism to set the trust cycle into motion. Without members' willingness to open up to each other, there will be no opportunities to give and receive empathy and experience belongingness and acceptance. Group therapists need to be skilled in both encouraging member self-disclosure, as well as encouraging members to validate and support self-disclosure when it happens (Chen & Rybak, 2018). These skills may involve well-timed prompts, gentle check-ins of quiet members, or group therapists modeling self-disclosure for members. If the group therapists have been thoughtful in the initial norming process, members will have some guidance about effective interpersonal behaviors to enact in a group.

Research suggests that group therapy outcomes are improved when group members are all engaging with empathy and curiosity and demonstrating a willingness to talk openly about culturally relevant issues (Grimes & Kivlighan, 2022; Kivlighan et al., 2019a; Owen et. al, 2016). Cultural comfort of the group has been positively correlated to BIPOC members' willingness to open up about themselves and their overall improvement in group therapy (Kivlighan et al., 2019b). Based on these findings, adopting, and integrating a MCO framework in group therapy is an important piece of the group cohesiveness puzzle.

Fear can be disruptive to the trust cycle because it can interfere with a person's willingness to be vulnerable, open, and trusting of others (Chen & Rybak, 2018). One way this fear can manifest is through cultural concealment, when someone intentionally hides culturally relevant aspects of self (Rigg & Kivlighan, 2022). BIPOC group members are more likely than White group members to conceal culturally salient aspects of themselves when they perceive the cultural comfort of the group to be low (Kivlighan et al., 2019b). BIPOC group members may suspect the cultural comfort of the group is low if the White members and group therapists are engaging in subtle behaviors meant to mask discomfort (e.g., overly positive affect, color neutral statements, intellectualizing; Kivlighan et al., 2019b). The presence of cultural discomfort, if unchecked, could stifle their willingness to open up and impair their connectedness to the group, which in turn will negatively impact their group therapy outcomes (Rigg & Kivlighan, 2022). Cultural comfort does not emerge immediately, and the presence of discomfort does not automatically indicate a lack of safety. If White domestic members seem uncomfortable with or outright avoidant of cultural conversations, group therapists can gently nudge those members to lean into their discomfort as a learning opportunity. Therapists able to skillfully navigate cultural discomfort dynamics, will create a new and potentially healing dynamic for BIPOC and ISC group members, where they get to witness their fellow White group members' growth in terms of cultural comfort. Thus, group therapists need to focus immediately on cultivating a safe and cohesive group space, to neutralize the impact of cultural concealment, cultural discomfort, and fear.

Performing Stage: Facilitating Growth and Healing.

In this stage, the group has reached peak maturity and is ready for powerful growth and healing. This growth and healing comes about in IP groups because of two primary group characteristics: a here-and-now focus and opportunities for experiential learning. This growth process is robust in comparison to change that comes about from simply talking about problems. Focusing on what is happening here-and-now allows IP group members the opportunity to get a "personal and direct experience of the interpersonal" in the present moment (Chen & Rybak, 2018, p. 19). The MCO framework integrates nicely with this growth process, as it involves developing a deeper understanding of self and others and increasing one's comfort zone. The growth that occurs in IP groups is an insight-building process that group therapists can facilitate by slowing the action down, inviting internal reflection (including written reflection), and eliciting interpersonal feedback from others. As members gain insight, they can then use the group space as a laboratory to try interacting differently with the benefit of real-time feedback (Chen & Rybak, 2018; Yalom & Leszcz, 2020).

The here-and-now and experiential dynamics of IP groups offer powerful healing opportunities through corrective emotional experiences. Corrective emotional experiences occur when interpersonal interactions between group members counter deeply held beliefs about self in relation to others—beliefs that are often informed by painful past relationship experiences (Yalom & Leszcz, 2020). With this type of emotional reality testing, a client's deeply held beliefs will transform. Within the context of relationships, cultural humility is transformative because it cultivates mutual respect, openness, empathy, understanding, and the experience of being seen (Foronda et al., 2016; Mosher et al., 2017). Orienting toward cultural humility in interactions with suffering members and then seizing cultural opportunities could be a powerful healing experience.

Dismantling Power Imbalance to Build Connections

As discussed previously, the literature has mostly focused on the benefits of group spaces composed of other international students where the focus is acculturation strategies and building community. As a group becomes more diverse and unstructured, it will resemble a microcosm of the interpersonal lives of the group members, as well as a reflection of cultural dynamics in larger society (Guth et al., 2019; Yalom & Leszcz, 2020). This means members will engage in potentially harmful behaviors, those behaviors will harm members, and members will have opportunities to experiment with new ways of interacting with others—all grist for the mill. Generalization of interpersonal learning is a fundamental goal for all IP groups (Guth et al., 2019). What this means is that members should ideally be able to apply what they learn in group to their lives outside of group. For ISC, this means they can experiment with taking up space in ways that they often do not outside of the group therapy space, where they might feel invisible or denigrated. For White students, whose privilege can keep them shielded from the experiences of less privileged groups, IP groups can challenge socialization based in neo-racism and offer opportunities to practice more affirming ways of interacting with others who are different from them.

It is not uncommon for ISC to only participate in conversations about news happening in the U.S. and to stifle their worries (i.e., cultural concealment) about, for instance, unrest in their home countries, anti-immigration policies, and xenophobia. Rather than remaining complicit or oblivious to cultural concealment, group therapists and members can create cultural opportunities for ISC to talk about these worries and concerns. ISC benefit in several ways when empowered to take space and show up fully, as opposed to concealing certain aspects of themselves. First, it normalizes, validates, supports, and empowers ISC to speak openly about their lives, which will decrease their sense of loneliness and isolation. Second, it has the potential to build awareness of privilege for domestic students, and provides an opportunity for them to engage with curiosity and compassion for ISC. Third, it promotes the full benefits of the MCO framework, reduces ethnocentric and cultural biases, and establishes a culturally affirmng and inclusive group climate. The ripple effects from this type of transformation extend outside of the group therapy space into the members' day-to-day interpersonal lives and beyond, slowly dismantling systemic power structures that are exclusive and damaging (Guth et al., 2019).

Impact of the Co-Therapy Relationship

Yalom and Leszcz (2020) emphasized the importance of *"how the therapist must be"* in group to enhance its effectiveness (p. 255). Within the context of the MCO framework, a therapist's orientation toward cultural humility, their level of cultural comfort, and willingness to initiate cultural opportunities are all positively correlated to the therapeutic alliance and their clients' therapeutic outcomes (Davis et al., 2018; Grimes & Kivlighan, 2022; Hook et al., 2013; Owen et al., 2016; Owen et al., 2011).

One of the co-authors of this chapter is a Caucasian U.S.-born female (KM) and the other is an Asian female with an international background (YL). Throughout our co-leading relationship, we have been intentional about adopting a MCO framework with each other. We have cultivated a good working relationship through mutual balance and support (in and out of group), as well as active and reflective communication—all important principles for a healthy co-leading relationship (Chen & Rybak, 2018). We have intentionally taken time outside of the group to talk openly about our own cultural contexts, debriefed the group action through a cultural lens—both in terms of the group process and our own reactions, and have given and received culturally relevant feedback to each other. Therefore, orienting toward multiculturalism is beneficial in the group therapists' relationship, just as it is beneficial in the relationships amongst group members and between group members and group therapists.

Just as group members project inaccurately onto each other, group members will also project onto the group therapists, i.e., transference (Yalom & Leszcz, 2020). This transference will, in part, be tied to the intersectionality of group therapists' and members' cultural identities. Successfully managing transference hinges on the members' ability to gain a deeper understanding of their true underlying reactions. Yalom and Leszcz (2020) suggest two ways of managing transference: 1) seeking out validation or invalidation of a member's belief from other group members; or 2) therapist self-disclosure and openness to reveal support or to challenge the belief. The MCO framework is congruent with these suggestions, as both of these approaches require the group therapists to be self-reflective (cultural humility), curious and open about others (cultural humility), comfortable with exploring culturally based transference (cultural comfort), and motivated to initiate those opportunities (cultural opportunities). For example, the group therapists noticed a pattern where a group member, who was international and biracial, would always talk to the White group therapist. This group therapist shared her observation and expressed curiosity to this member in a non-judgmental way, which led to the member self-disclosing her fear of being judged by the Asian therapist as "not Asian enough." The Asian group therapist revealed her genuine connection with this member, and adopted a stance of emotional equanimity (meaning openness, curiosity, and non-judgment) and invited the member to say more. The member shared that she was biracial and that her father was from Germany and mother from mainland China. She was raised in Germany and closely connected to her German, but not Chinese, heritage, under the influence of her abusive mother. This cultural opportunity allowed this member to open up more about her family trauma and the challenges of her cultural identity development, which led to a rich conversation for other members about family dynamics, transference and countertransference within the group, and shame and guilt. In the termination session, the member acknowledged that her prior belief had been disconfirmed and the genuine connection with the Asian group therapist was a significant corrective experience for her.

Teaching or Case Examples

In this section, we will present a group case example to show how the MCO framework can play out in an IP group interaction. In this case example we will show both the growth and healing processes at play through the lens of the MCO framework. Through this clinical example we hope to bring to life these complex concepts with the hopes of offering practical intervention strategies/techniques.

Shifting from Cultural Imposition to Cultural Humility

In the third session of an IP group focused on family trauma, the session started as usual with a brief check-in. During check-in, Anna, an ISC from Nigeria, talked about having a difficult week after talking to her mother. Once check-ins were over, Joe, a White domestic student, expressed curiosity and invited Anna to talk more about the conversation with her mother. What transpired between these two members was a lesson in cultural imposition vs cultural humility.

Self-Disclosure

Anna expressed gratitude for the invitation. Anna talked about her mother being manipulative, talking about frequent guilt-trips, criticisms of Anna, and ultimatums. Anna stated that her most recent conversation was more of the same, but this time Anna got upset and raised her voice to her mother. Her mother's reaction was to shame Anna for being a bad daughter and to threaten to disown her if she ever raises her voice again. Anna stated that she was extremely upset but finally backed down and apologized to her mother. She acknowledged to the group that she was feeling both ashamed and resentful. She ended by saying that she wished she could cut all ties with her mother but said that is not possible. Anna was tearful throughout this disclosure. Group therapists could sense the heaviness of Anna's suffering and noticed the group was focused on her with rapt attention—looking intently at her, leaning in, stillness. One group therapist said to the group:

> "I can tell that many of you are impacted by what Anna just shared. I'm curious what thoughts or feelings you were experiencing as you listened to Anna." *[eliciting validation and empathy from group members]*

Cultural Imposition

In response to the group therapist's prompt, Joe spoke up and expressed anger for how Anna had been treated. He went on to express his belief that Anna should cut off contact from her mother because she does not deserve to be treated that way. He added that she has nothing to feel ashamed about.

Cultural Concealment.

Anna offered a half-smile and said "thanks" to Joe and did not say anything else. Group therapists sensed a shift in Anna and in the atmosphere in the group. One group therapist said:

> "It seems like you (to Joe) were trying to connect with Anna, and I'm wondering how what Joe said landed with you, Anna."
> *[group therapists eliciting IP feedback]*

Anna responded with appreciation for Joe's perspective, but again seemed guarded or withdrawn. A group therapist made this observation:

> "I'm noticing that something has shifted for you Anna—you seem more guarded or withdrawn since Joe offered his reaction to you. I wonder if his desire to connect did not land as intended."
> *[process illumination, expressing curiosity, inviting self-disclosure]*

IP Feedback.

Anna acknowledged the group therapist was correct. The group therapist redirected Anna to speak directly to Joe. She told Joe that his reaction made her bristle and acknowledged that she did not want to tell him that for fear of upsetting him. The group therapist responded:

> "Thank you so much for letting us know, Anna. Joe, Anna just let you know that your intention to connect missed her. How are you feeling hearing that?"

Self-Reflection and Cultural Humility

Joe expressed appreciation for Anna's honesty and apologized for offending her. He explained that he cut off his abusive father and it felt liberating to him, so he wanted to offer that as a solution to Anna. He said that he now realizes that just because it worked for him does not mean it will work for Anna. He then expressed compassion for Anna, acknowledging that it must be hard to have such a strained relationship with her mother. In an expression of curiosity, he inquired about how her values made it difficult to cut ties with her mother.

Cultural Opportunity

Anna talked to the group about her cultural heritage and socialization around family and obligation to family. She indicated that these cultural values are an important part of her identity and something on which she does not want to compromise. Group leaders invited Anna to elaborate on her cultural values either in English or her native language (cultural humility), she shared an idiom "Iza ka mma na Nne Ji" which means that the wisdom is best shared through bloodiness and the importance of training children through parents, grandparents, and their village. In response to this, group members expressed both understanding and acceptance of her values, and worried for her well-being.

Corrective Emotional Experience

This interaction ended with Anna stating that she rarely expresses herself honestly like she did with Joe. She appreciated that Joe listened to her rather than yelling at her, like her mother would have. She wondered if she should start being more open with her feelings moving forward.

Discussion

This example started with Joe taking a genuine interest in hearing more from Anna about her check-in, a characteristic of cultural humility. Anna was grateful for Joe's interest, which seemed to reassure her that she was safe to say more. Her sense of safety and trust in the group is evident in her expression of shame and tears. Group therapists read the non-verbals of the other group members and could tell they were highly engaged. Group leaders prompted the group members to check in and tell Anna about their feelings, to elicit validation, empathy, and here-and-now self-awareness.

Joe's response to Anna seemed well-intentioned but, ultimately, had the unintended consequence of shutting down the process. The group leaders recognized that Joe's response to Anna demonstrated characteristics in opposition to cultural humility, specifically making assumptions, believing he knew more than he actually did, and inadvertently disempowering Anna—a cultural imposition. Understandably, Anna's presentation shifted from open to closed, alerting the group leaders to the possibility Anna was engaging in cultural concealment.

As highlighted in the previous section, an interaction like this could be reenacting experiences Anna has in her daily life, and if not attended to, could cause a significant rupture between Anna the rest of the group. This kind of rupture interferes with the benefits and therapeutic benefits of group, for Anna, for other ISC, and, possibly, for the entire group. To avoid this, group therapists highlighted the shift in the group atmosphere and invited Anna to give Joe interpersonal feedback. Their first attempt was unsuccessful, so the group therapists tried again by making direct observations of Anna's behavior and explicitly highlighting the potential rupture. This second attempt was successful, giving Anna an opportunity to voice her genuine reactions, an opportunity that she may not feel safe seizing in her daily life. Because this group was still relatively early in its development (session 3), group leaders were intentional about directing the action between Joe and Anna, to ensure that they both were listening to each other and were given a chance to speak.

Now we see the shift from cultural imposition to cultural humility in Joe. His response to Anna was respectful, self-reflective, compassionate, open to perspective, and curious to learn more. Anna shifted from closed and guarded back to openness. She seemed both reassured and encouraged by Joe's curiosity, which facilitated a cultural opportunity for Anna to describe her cultural heritage and socialization. Anna's openness allowed members to understand her complicated perspective on her mother more fully, which allowed them to express their own genuine worry for Anna along with their understanding and acceptance of Anna's point of view. The cultural humility that developed in this interaction paved the way for a corrective emotional experience, where Anna got to express her displeasure with Joe, something that has felt impossible for her to do in other circumstances of her life (e.g., with her mother). This opened Anna up to the possibility that, perhaps, others outside of her family would be more receptive to her feelings—the corrective emotional experience.

Ethical Considerations

MCO as a Matter of Justice and Non-Maleficence

Adopting a MCO framework aligns with ethical guidelines for group therapy. According to Logan (2020), "Therapists who have not undergone formalized inquiry into the questions of othering may, in fact, be working outside of their scope of practice" (p. 29). When we work outside of the bounds of our competence, we are at risk of harming those we are trying to help. Additionally, group therapists are bound to the ethical principle of justice, in this case making sure that group therapy spaces truly serve all group members, so everyone benefits equally (Brabender & MacNair-Semands, 2022). MCO offers a helpful approach to avoid the harm of othering and the injustice of exclusivity because it involves both critical self-reflection and openness and curiosity to learning from others (Mosher et al., 2017). Additionally, cultural humility is a lifelong journey of growth and discovery and an intentional shift in language from cultural competence. This distinction is important because cultural competence might imply that one might achieve total competence and potential mastery (Owen et al., 2011; Tervalon & Murray-García, 1998).

As mentioned previously, it is not uncommon for the perceived limitations or challenges of ISC to be over-emphasized when considering the needs of this group (Lee & Rice, 2007; Yao et al., 2018). While the intention might be good (i.e., beneficence—to help relieve suffering), this can also do harm, for instance over-pathologizing ISC, perpetuating stereotypes and misinformation, and perpetrating microaggressions and discrimination. Instead, we encourage group therapists to use the three pillars of MCO to attend to both the needs and strengths of ISC (e.g., strong community ties, resources, multilingual competence, life and cultural experience, self-determination).

Another ethical consideration related to avoiding harm and enacting justice involves the group therapist's role in harmful or destructive group interactions. The "AGPA Guidelines for Creating Affirming Group Experiences" (Aguirre et al., n.d.) recommends group therapists and/or members use microinterventions in response to microaggressions. According to Sue and colleagues (2019), the purpose of a microintervention is to validate, affirm, support, connect, and reassure the target of a microaggression. The authors describe four goals with these statements, "(a) make the invisible visible, (b) disarm the microaggression, (c educate the perpetrator, and (d) seek external reinforcement or support" (p. 128). If the group therapist is the perpetrator of a microaggression, Aguirre and colleagues (n.d.) emphasize the importance for therapists to avoid defending themselves, take responsibility and engage with curiosity, apologize sincerely, express appreciation for the feedback, and continue the learning process. If left unaddressed, microaggressions perpetrated against ISC can do harm and interfere with their growth and healing.

Ethical Considerations Relevant to ISC

Ethical considerations that seem to transcend culture may actually be incredibly culturally relevant. For instance, group therapists may need to adapt their informed consent practice for international students, who may have limited knowledge of group therapy and may be limited in their English proficiency (Dipeolu et al., 2007; Walker & Conyne, 2007; Yakunina et al., 2011). Pre-group screening appointments, as well as clear and concise informed consent documentation, are crucial to ensure IS understand their rights and what to expect. ISC may have an additional concern about feeling like an outsider in a group of predominantly White people. Group therapists should assess this concern and be ready to discuss what they know about the racial and ethnic composition of the group, along with group therapists' intentions to attend to cultural factors.

Privacy and confidentiality is another seemingly basic ethical arena that is more complicated with international students for a couple of reasons. First, one's understanding of privacy and confidentiality varies across cultures, so, to use an ethical approach, group therapists must spend time answering questions and ensuring international students know when confidentiality and privacy rules apply and when they do not apply (Yakunina et al., 2011). Second, confidentiality and privacy become more complicated when group members' lives intersect outside of groups (e.g., being in the same class or student organization; tight-knit community). For ISC in particular, acculturative stress, neo-racism, and isolation may motivate them to stay in communities of people with shared or similar backgrounds (Johnson & Sandhu, 2007).

Implications for Training and Practice

We believe that cultural considerations should become a universal and intentional approach to training and education in group therapy, as well as the practice of group therapy itself. In other words, a MCO should become a foundational approach to all types of group therapy, not just groups set up as affinity spaces for marginalized communities.

If You Start with Cultural Humility, the Rest Will Come

Adopting the MCO framework must start with cultural humility, which, in turn, starts with critical self-reflection. This includes reflection on important similar and different identities between therapist and group members, and how those identities will affect all the IP dynamics in groups (Mosher et al., 2017). For instance, one author (KM) could ask herself, "As a White, cisgender, American woman, how do my intersecting identities shape my worldview, create knowledge gaps that might emerge in diverse spaces, contribute to power imbalances, and potentially impede the therapeutic alliance? What do I take for granted when I walk around the world being a native English speaker, being White, being born and raised in the United States of America?" The other author (YL) could self-reflect, "As a woman of Color with an international background, how can I increase my level of consciousness in cultural countertransference? How can I transform my personal encounters with racism, identity formation, and immigration challenges to effectively promote support and advocacy for ISC?" These deeply personal reflection questions reveal the lifelong, transformative nature of cultural humility. Cultural humility is not a set of skills or competencies that one learns in one or two training sessions. Instead, it is an other-oriented worldview that requires deep and ongoing reflection and critique of the boundaries of one's own knowledge.

A therapist's orientation toward cultural humility should be driven by an intrinsic motivation to attune to cultural dynamics happening in group therapy spaces, to seek out skills and strategies for cultivating culturally inclusive and curious group therapy spaces, and to make the world more inclusive for everyone. As therapists cultivate their own cultural humility, they also grow more resilient and at ease with cultural issues, and, thus, more willing to engage with clients in this way. This process lets go of the pressure for the therapist to be a "knower" of culture or the expert on their clients, which reenacts harmful power imbalances that ISC encounter in their daily lives (Bemak & Chung, 2015).

Education is key to integrating a MCO framework into one's practice and into training programs. We advocate for programs training mental health practitioners to integrate the MCO framework throughout all aspects of their respective curricula. We also recommend experienced and inexperienced group therapists seek out formal, interactive, and intensive culturally oriented educational opportunities. Ideally this education will be interactive and experiential, including space to reflect internally and openly with others to facilitate deep, personal learning. These experiences should be as intensive and immersive as possible, as opposed to brief one-at-a-time experiences, to give time for the break-down and digestion of complex material. We also recommend group therapists participate in culturally oriented interpersonal process groups. Training groups like this can offer affinity spaces for support and healing around marginalized identities, or growth-oriented spaces for reflection on privileged identities. In addition to more formal sources of education, we recommend group therapists engage in self-study and more informal cultural opportunities, such as reading books, watching movies, tuning into the local and global news, and immersing oneself in culturally related activities. Chen and Rybak (2018) strongly encourage group therapists to engage in reflective writing practices to develop cultural humility, from both a personal (e.g., one's feelings, thoughts, reactions) and a critical perspective (e.g., IP group process and dynamics).

In addition to education, we also advocate for implementing mechanisms to collect client feedback in group therapy spaces. Apart from the therapeutic benefits, collecting client feedback also fits into a social justice framework by: 1) dismantling potential power imbalances and elevating the client's voice; 2) increasing insight for both therapists and clients; and 3) promoting on-going self-reflection (Minieri et al., 2015). While a number of systems exist for collecting client feedback, we want to highlight one in particular, Multicultural Orientation Inventory—Group Version (MCO-G), also recommended by MacNair-Semands and Whittingham (2023) in their book. The MCO-G was developed by Kivlighan and colleagues (2019a) to measure group members' perceptions of the presence of cultural humility, cultural comfort, and cultural opportunities at the group level.

Conclusion

ISC are a highly marginalized, misunderstood, and culturally diverse population. They have a wide range of strengths and lived experiences that contribute positively to U.S. higher educational institutions and larger society. Additionally, they also experience a great deal of stress and difficulty stemming from acculturation stress and neo-racism. Participating in IP groups can be an activating experience for ISC, as groups can become microcosms of the group members' interpersonal lives and of larger society. For IP groups to *also* be a healing and growth-oriented experience, we strongly recommend group therapists adopt a MCO framework for all group therapy experiences they lead, since every group, even the most homogeneous ones, are heterogeneous and diverse in many other ways (Yalom & Leszcz, 2020).

References

Aguirre, M. S., Belcher Platt, A., Brookens, L., Brooks, S., Dehili, V., Evans, M., Freedman, W., Gentuso, S., Gitterman, P., Griffin, L., Haen, C., Horner, P., Ribeiro, M., Sheppard, T., Steiner, A., Turner, M. M., Klein, L., Murphy-Swiller, L., & Williams, L. (n.d.). *Guidelines for creating affirming group experiences*. American Group Psychotherapy Association. https://agpa.org/home/media/social-issue-policy-resolutions/agpa-guidelines-for-creating-affirming-group-experiences.

American Psychological Association. (2017). *Ethical principles of psychologists and code of conduct* (2002, amended effective June 1, 2010, and January 1, 2017). www.apa.org/ethics/code/index.html.

Bateman, A. W., Fonagy, P., & Campbell, C. (2018). Mentalization-based treatment. In W. J. Livesley & R. Larstone (Eds), *Handbook of personality disorders: Theory, research, and treatment* (2nd Edition, pp. 541–554). Guilford Press.

Bemak, F. & Chung, R. C. Y. (2015). Critical issues in international group counseling. *The Journal for Specialists in Group Work, 40*(1), 6–21. https://doi.org/10.1080/01933922.2014.992507.

Blum, L. (2015). Race and class categories and subcategories in educational thought and research. *Theory and Research in Education, 13*(1), 87–104. https://doi.org/10.1177/1477878514562687.

Brabender, V. & MacNair-Semands, R. (2022). *The ethics of group psychotherapy: Principles and practical strategies*. Routledge. https://doi.org/10.4324/9781003105527.

Chen, M. & Rybak, C. (2018). *Group leadership skills: Interpersonal process in group counseling and therapy* (2nd Edition). Sage Publications, Inc. https://doi.org/10.4135/9781071800980.

Davis, D. E., DeBlaere, C., Owen, J., Hook, J. N., Rivera, D. P., Choe, E., Van Tongeren, D. R., Worthington, E. L., Jr., & Placeres, V. (2018). The multicultural orientation framework: A narrative review. *Psychotherapy, 55*(1), 89–100. https://doi.org/10.1037/pst0000160.

Davis, D. E., Worthington, E. L., Hook, J. N., Emmons, R. A., Hill, P. C., Bollinger, R. A., & Van Tongeren, D. R. (2013). Humility and the development and repair of social bonds: Two longitudinal studies. *Self and Identity, 12*(1), 58–77. https://doi.org/10.1080/15298868.2011.636509.

Delgado-Romero, E. A. & Wu, Y.-C. (2010). Asian international students in counseling programs: A group intervention to promote social justice. *The Journal for Specialists in Group Work, 35*(3), 290–298. https://doi.org/10.1080/01933922.2010.492896.

Dipeolu, A., Kang, J., & Cooper, C. (2007). Support group for international students: A counseling center's experience. *Journal of College Student Psychotherapy, 22*(1), 63–74. https://doi.org/10.1300/J035v22n01_05.

Foronda, C., Baptiste, D. L., Reinholdt, M. M., & Ousman, K. (2016). Cultural humility: A concept analysis. *Journal of Transcultural Nursing, 27*(3), 210–217. https://doi.org/10.1177/1043659615592677.

George Mwangi, C. A. & English, S. (2017). Being Black (and) immigrant students: When race, ethnicity, and nativity collide. *International Journal of Multicultural Education, 19*(2), 100–130. https://doi.org/10.18251/ijme.v19i2.1317.

Glass, C. R., Heng, T. T., & Hou, M. (2022). Intersections of identity and status in international students' perceptions of culturally engaging campus environments. *International Journal of Intercultural Relations, 89*, 19–29. https://doi.org/10.1016/j.ijintrel.2022.05.003

Grimes, J. L. & Kivlighan, D. M. (2022). Whose multicultural orientation matters most? Examining additive and compensatory effects of the group's and leader's multicultural orientation in group therapy. *Group Dynamics: Theory, Research, and Practice, 26*(1), 58–70. https://doi.org/10.1037/gdn0000153.

Guth, L. J., Pollard, B. L., Nitza, A., Puig, A., Chan, C. D., Singh, A. A., & Bailey, H. (2019). Ten strategies to intentionally use group work to transform hate, facilitate courageous conversations, and enhance community building. *The Journal for specialists in group work, 44*(1), 3–24. https://doi.org/10.1080/01933922.2018.1561778.

Hook, J. N., Davis, D. E., Owen, J., Worthington, E. L., Jr., & Utsey, S. O. (2013). Cultural humility: Measuring openness to culturally diverse clients. *Journal of Counseling Psychology, 60*(3), 353–366. https://doi.org/10.1037/a0032595.

Johnson, L. R. & Sandhu, D. S. (2007). Isolation, adjustment, and acculturation issues of international students: Intervention strategies for counselors. In H. D. Singaravelu & M. Pope (Eds.), *A handbook for counseling international students in the United States* (pp. 13–35). American Counseling Association.

Kivlighan, D. M. III, Adams, M. C., Drinane, J. M., Tao, K. W., & Owen, J. (2019a). Construction and validation of the Multicultural Orientation Inventory—Group Version. *Journal of Counseling Psychology, 66*(1), 45–55. https://doi.org/10.1037/cou0000294.

Kivlighan, D. M. III, Drinane, J. M., Tao, K. W., Owen, J., & Liu, W. M. (2019b). The detrimental effect of fragile groups: Examining the role of cultural comfort for group therapy members of Color. *Journal of Counseling Psychology, 66*(6), 763–770. https://doi.org/10.1037/cou0000352.

Lee, J. J. & Rice, C. (2007) Welcome to America? International student perceptions of discrimination. *Higher Education, 53,* 381–409. https://doi-org.libproxy.wustl.edu/10.1007/s10734-005-4508-3.

Logan, G. (2020). The shadows of liberty. In M. D. Ribeiro (Ed.), *Examining social identities and diversity issues in group therapy: Knocking at the boundaries* (pp. 24–37). Routledge. https://doi.org/10.4324/9780429022364.

MacNair-Semands, R., & Whittingham, M. (Eds). (2023). *Group psychotherapy assessment and practice: A measurement-based care approach.* Routledge. https://doi.org/10.4324/9781003255482.

Minieri, A. M., Reese, R. J., Miserocchi, K. M., & Pascale-Hague, D. (2015). Using client feedback in training of future counseling psychologists: An evidence-based and social justice practice. *Counselling Psychology Quarterly, 28*(3), 305–323. https://doi.org/10.1080/09515070.2015.1055236.

Mosher, D. K., Hook, J. N., Captari, L. E., Davis, D. E., DeBlaere, C., & Owen, J. (2017). Cultural humility: A therapeutic framework for engaging diverse clients. *Practice Innovations, 2*(4), 221–233. https://doi.org/10.1037/pri0000055.

National Association of Foreign Student Advisers: Association of International Educators. (2020). *Losing talent 2020: An economic and foreign policy risk America can't ignore.* www.nafsa.org/sites/default/files/media/document/nafsa-losing-talent.pdf.

Open Doors. (2022). *Leading places of origin of international students* [Infographic]. Opendoorsdata.org. https://opendoorsdata.org/data/international-students/enrollment-trends.

Owen, J. J., Tao, K., Leach, M. M., & Rodolfa, E. (2011). Clients' perceptions of their psychotherapists' multicultural orientation. *Psychotherapy, 48*(3), 274–282. https://doi.org/10.1037/a0022065

Owen, J., Tao, K. W., Drinane, J. M., Hook, J., Davis, D. E., & Kune, N. F. (2016). Client perceptions of therapists' multicultural orientation: Cultural (missed) opportunities and cultural humility. *Professional Psychology: Research and Practice, 47*(1), 30–37. https://doi.org/10.1037/pro0000046.

PettyJohn, M. E., Tseng, C.-F., & Blow, A. J. (2020). Therapeutic utility of discussing therapist/client intersectionality in treatment: When and how? *Family Process, 59*(2), 313–327. https://doi.org/10.1111/famp.12471.

Ribeiro, M. D. (2020). Social identities explored in therapy groups. In M. D. Ribeiro (Ed.), *Examining social identities and diversity issues in group therapy: Knocking at the boundaries* (pp. 78–92). Routledge. https://doi.org/10.4324/9780429022364.

Rigg, T. & Kivlighan, M. (2022). Examining between-group and within-group cultural concealment in group therapy. *Professional Psychology: Research and Practice, 53*(3), 244–252. https://doi.org/10.1037/pro0000458.

Sue, D. W., Alsaidi, S., Awad, M. N., Glaeser, E., Calle, C. Z., & Mendez, N. (2019). Disarming racial microaggressions: Microintervention strategies for targets, White allies, and bystanders. *American Psychologist, 74*(1), 128–142. https://doi.org/10.1037/amp0000296.

Tervalon, M. & Murray-García, J. (1998). Cultural humility versus cultural competence: A critical distinction in defining physician training outcomes in multicultural education. *Journal of Health Care for the Poor and Underserved, 9*(2), 117–125. https://doi.org/10.1353/hpu.2010.0233.

Tuckman, B. W. (1965). Developmental sequence in small groups. *Psychological Bulletin, 63*(6), 384–399. https://doi.org/10.1037/h0022100.

Walker, L. A., & Conyne, R. K. (2007). Group work with international students. In H. D. Singaravelu & M. Pope (Eds), *A handbook for counseling international students in the United States* (pp. 13–35). American Counseling Association.

Yakunina, E. S., Weigold, I. K., & McCarthy, A. S. (2011). Group counseling with international students: Practical, ethical, and cultural considerations. *Journal of College Student Psychotherapy, 25*(1), 67–78. https://doi.org/10.1080/87568225.2011.532672.

Yalom, I. D. & Leszcz, M. (2020). *The theory and practice of group psychotherapy* (6th Edition). Basic Books.

Yang, P. (2020). China in the global field of international student mobility: an analysis of economic, human and symbolic capitals. *Compare: A Journal of Comparative and International Education. 52*(3), 1–19. https://doi.org/10.1080/03057925.2020.1764334.

Yao, C. W., George Mwangi, C. A., & Malaney Brown, V. K. (2018). Exploring the intersection of transnationalism and critical race theory: A critical race analysis of international students in the United States. *Race Ethnicity and Education 22*(1), 38–58. https://doi.org/10.1080/13613324.2018.1497968.

Yau, T. Y. (2004). Guidelines for facilitating groups with international college students. In J. L. DeLucia-Waack, D. A. Gerrity, C. R. Kalodner, & M. T. Riva (Eds), *Handbook of group counseling and psychotherapy* (pp. 253–264). Sage Publications. https://doi.org/10.4135/9781452229683.n18.

Yeo, H. J. T., Mendenhall, R., Harwood, S. A., & Huntt, M. B. (2019). Asian international student and Asian American student: Mistaken identity and racial microaggressions. *Journal of International Students, 9*(1), 39–65. https://doi.org/10.32674/jis.v9i1.278.

Yoon, E., Chang, C.-T., Kim, S., Clawson, A., Clearly, S. E., Hansen, M., Bruner, J. P., Chan, T. K., & Gomes, A. M. (2013). A meta-analysis of acculturation/enculturation and mental health. *Journal of Counseling Psychology, 60*(1), 15–30. https://doi.org/10.1037/a0030652.

4 Hidden Diversity

The Invisible Oppressor of Classism

Cindy Miller Aron and Sydney Marie LeFay

Conceptual Framework

Classism, defined as a belief that a person's social or economic station in society determines their value in that society, is an under-explored and under-acknowledged bias in group therapy practice and training. Studies reveal that psychotherapists often fail to identify three factors affecting socioeconomic status (SES)—occupation, income, and education—and also fail to identify subjective social status (SSS) as a component of class identity (Cook, 2019; Demakakos, 2008). Understanding the distinction of social class and socioeconomic status in ourselves as clinicians as well as our clients are crucial variables in the development of multicultural competence. Class identity broadly intersects with other marginalized identities, including racial, gender, sexual, and disability status. This intersectionality increases the interpersonal complexity of relationships between therapists, individual clients, and group members. In this chapter we explore the impact of classism in the group therapy setting, using sociological conceptualizations of class, case examples, and a review of relevant literature on classism in group psychotherapy.

All individuals, therapists, and clients, hold their own unique class identity and related biases. Examination of class biases is a necessary point of self-reflection for group psychotherapists in practice and in training settings, where a lack of sensitivity to classism can lead to erasure of important aspects of identity and ultimately a lack of attunement to the needs of clients (Smith, 2005). Class-related cultural transference and countertransference within the therapeutic relationship can be important components of a developing working alliance (Gelso & Mohr, 2001).

In exploring classism, we must clearly define the nature of class identity. Social class is defined as a combination of a person's SES, which is an easier and more objective metric of class, along with subjective social status SSS, referring to a person's perception of their relative position in social hierarchy (Cook, 2019; Demakakos et al., 2008). As previously defined, SES includes the three factors of income, occupation, and education, all of which can change over the course of a lifetime (Cook, 2019).

A person's SSS is culturally bound and may contain a multitude of factors leading to a person's perceived class standing. This encompasses class-cultural beliefs, attitudes, values, access to resources, level of education, occupation, social behaviors, immigration country and/or status (rural, urban, or suburban) and potentially a multitude of other subtle factors. Examples of SSS affecting a person's experience of the world may include expectations and judgments of what is "success" or "failure" in life. Depending on a person's class perceptions, the achievement of attending a trade school and obtaining an apprenticeship may be

DOI: 10.4324/9781003455783-6

viewed as highly respectable and desirable, or alternatively, seen as a failure to achieve a "white collar" profession, depending on a person's classist biases.

Identity-related complications can emerge when socioeconomic status variables change. Individuals may identify and be identified as part of one social class group, yet have a fundamental, internal experience of being part of another group. For example, as a result of educational achievement, an individual may be viewed and identify as middle class, and yet also feel internally as if they are from a lower socioeconomic class, owing to the socioeconomic status of their family of origin. This can also pose complications for therapists who can bring assumptions and bias to the therapy room. Beliefs are maintained interpersonally through perceptions about social class, hierarchy, and nuanced judgment about perceived life chances, opportunities, and prospects (Choi, 2018). Additionally, social media and entertainment venues such as television create images that are often static, not changing over time, perpetuating stereotypes, and bias.

Intersectionality

Classism impacts systemically oppressed identities in a variety of ways. There is substantial evidence supporting the intersection between class and racial identity, where the wealth divides particularly between white, black, and Latinx populations remains stark, with an estimated $236,500 gap in median net worth between black and white families in the United States (Shapiro, 2013). People of color and women are both over-represented amongst those living in poverty, with women 40 percent more likely to experience poverty than men (Smith, 2008). LGBTQIA+ individuals are more likely to experience or be significantly impacted by a lower socioeconomic status (SES) than their heterosexual counterparts, and transgender individuals are four times as likely to report income less than $10,000 per year (American Psychological Association, 2002). People with disabilities are also known to be disproportionately of low SES and with lower levels of education (Smith, 2008). Disability status historically has been viewed as a defect rather than a difference. As a result, disability status has not been widely recognized as a multicultural concern. This is particularly notable since disability status can also change over a lifetime (Taylor, 2018). The intersectionality of class, race, disability status, gender, and sexual identity contributes to a societal tendency to dismiss or silence the voices of those from a lower SES. Systemic oppression is amplified by the intersection of these marginalized identities.

Microaggressions

Social class microaggressions such as 'you don't look like you grew up poor,' 'be proud of what you have overcome,' 'everyone should be like you,' 'you are a role model for your people,' and so on, denigrate and disrespect people who have non-dominant social class identities (Cook, 2019). The concept of The American Dream can perpetuate the "myth of a classless society" through the powerful belief that working hard allows all individuals to achieve whatever they wish (Newton, 2010). This United States myth goes largely unchallenged. The notion of meritocracy (i.e., hard work leads to success) is appealing and can relieve those in positions of privilege who experience a sense of discomfort with their privilege. The continued disparity in wealth in the United States and other countries, as well as limited class mobility, challenges this myth of the American Dream being held up as a standard. A capitalist society can be viewed as dependent on the existence of an underclass, primarily promoting the value of a broad middle class, which is viewed as holding the greatest cultural power (McDowell et al., 2013).

This myth of a classless society conflicts with the notion that social class tends to be understood from a hierarchical perspective. Society values occupations based upon socioeconomic status variables of education and income. Societal roles tend to be understood from a hierarchical perspective from low to high social class, often on a scale of lower to higher power and privilege. Opportunity is often tied to income. The binds inherent in this unintended caste system perpetuate the literal and psychological experience of societal members in each class. Hierarchical microaggressions are so common that they go unnoticed and/or unaddressed. Proclamations like 'why be a teacher when you have the intellect to be a doctor,' 'the military is a good place for those without other options,' 'I only have a master's degree,' and other similar judgments may be seen as "normalized" by those in positions of privilege.

Social systems such as communities, families, therapy groups inherently move towards the preservation of homeostasis, which can subtly affect an individuals' tendency to wish to share a sense of identity, rather than highlighting differences (Cook, 2020). Our brains naturally engage in a scan for likeness (Cook, 2020). This neurobiological inclination sets the stage for the ideology that the United States is a 'melting pot' with equal ingredients put together into one. It maintains the illusion that the middle class includes most people, and/or is accessible to most people and holds the most cultural power. When people are in a position of privilege this allows a 'freedom' to believe that they do not engage in microaggressions and, or hold different kinds of biases (Cook, 2020).

Group Interventions

While the literature contains some useful information on the impact of classism in individual psychotherapy, there is a dearth of literature on the impact of social class in group psychotherapy specifically. Psychotherapy training and research rarely address issues of class, often focusing on individualistic assessments which may miss larger socioeconomic factors in a client's well-being (McEvoy et.al., 2021). Issues of class may be magnified in the group setting where the examination of differences in identity is amplified by the nature of the modality. This does provide an opportunity for identification and exploration of this invisible 'ism.' It is essential to managing our biases, to understand the ways that ones' SES and SSS affect how we identify ourselves, but also how we come to identify others. Therapists, like others in society, are subjected to implicit messages emphasizing individual achievement regardless of a person's background, sidelining or trivializing the impact of systemic forces on a person's opportunities and identity. As group leaders who are in a role of professional power, there can be unintentional maintenance of these hierarchies for those who are blind to issues of classism.

The conceptual complexity of classism highlights the importance of exploring class-related bias in group therapy settings, including member-to-member, member-to-leader, and leader-to-member challenges that may arise. Here we will consider the impact of systemic class-based discrimination on the group psychotherapy profession as a whole, recognizing that pathways to group psychotherapy training often favor therapists from more privileged class backgrounds, creating potential gaps in understanding between the therapists and group participants as well as supervisors and supervisees.

Therapists' Educational Background

The journey to obtaining clinical training and certifications presents a multitude of barriers to practitioners with less class privilege and leads to a concentration of therapists from more privileged SES backgrounds (AAMC, 2008; Ballinger & Wright, 2007; Christophers et al., 2022; Dougall & Schwartz, 2011). Where most psychotherapy professions require graduate coursework, it is notable that in a longitudinal study of student achievement relative to family SES, approximately 14 percent of individuals from a low SES go on to complete a bachelor's degree or higher, while 29 percent of individuals with moderate SES and 60 percent of individuals from high SES backgrounds will obtain a higher-level degree (National Center for Education Statistics, 2015). The likelihood of successful completion of a degree after enrollment increases proportionally relative to SES background, likely related to a variety of factors including access to resources, need to contribute to the family of origin, and less guidance from their families (Titus, 2006).

These gaps in academic attainment based on family SES alone create a substantial demographic gap between therapists and many of their clients, as well as between disadvantaged trainees and their mentors who are likely to come from a higher SES background. Reduced access to quality primary education, restricted economic freedom to pursue degrees of higher education, lack of representation in the field, and social or familial expectations regarding occupation present challenges to increasing the number of therapists from more diverse socioeconomic strata (Yan & Gai, 2022). Research on the experiences of therapists from low SES while in training is sparse, perhaps as a function of the lack of representation of people from low SES in positions of power.

Classism Dynamics in Groups

For group leaders coming from a place of relative privilege, there may be gaps in understanding group members whose social class substantially differs from their own. The broader social tendency to minimize discussion of class may reinforce a leader's unintentional collusion with silencing important issues related to class in group discourse. Conversely, group leaders with a history of prior class-related disadvantages may receive various projections from group members and colleagues alike who presume a background of privilege, owing to the therapist's current social status. Trainees may struggle to describe their experience of class-related discrimination and bias given a lack of discussion during training. A trainee from a disadvantaged background may feel pressure to avoid volunteering their own differences in environments where their peers and mentors are often of a relatively privileged class background.

Issues of classism are highly relevant in the supervision and training setting. Increasing diversity in any demographic, whether class, racial, gender, or sexual identity diversity, hinges on developing environments that are welcoming to people from these identities (Wiley & Manstead, 2018). Among many complex barriers to achieving professional status and continuing to contribute in academic spheres, the sense of not belonging or being out of place is an important consideration for people of a lower SES (Wiley & Manstead, 2018). Encouraging the involvement of mentors from diverse backgrounds is one important step towards helping a trainee "see" themselves in their aspired profession, however, this may be difficult in fields where senior practitioners are overwhelmingly from a particular demographic (in this case, people raised in a primarily middle- or upper-class status). The ideal circumstance in which trainees are exposed to senior practitioners from a wide variety of backgrounds may not be immediately possible in any given institution, and in any case, all practitioners who choose to be involved in mentorship must be prepared to support the development of trainees whose backgrounds differ from their own. Among the many resilience factors thought to contribute to academic success in disadvantaged students, a harmonious or positive, close relationship with teachers is a modifiable factor institutions and mentors foster (Yan & Gai, 2022). Conversations about gender or racial identity are still developing on institutional levels, and in a similar vein, broad discussion of other 'isms' including classism has much room for expansion.

Cultural and institutional classism are embedded in the social structures that support the practice of psychotherapy. The invisibility of class bias makes it easier to minimize or ignore, subjugating the individuals who are the unwitting recipients. The "American Dream" can perpetuate the "myth of a classless society" through the powerful belief that working hard allows individuals to achieve whatever they wish to (Newton, 2010). Additionally, classism does not exist in a categorical way, it exists on a continuum, making it difficult for individuals to figure out where they are on this continuum. Objective standards like socioeconomic status can place a person in one spot on this continuum and social class identification can locate an individual on another. This is complicated by the murkiness of class boundaries in the United States. Individuals from backgrounds that are considered less privileged internalize this sense of their 'station in life' without appreciating how deeply integrated it is into their sense of self-value and power. On a subjective level, beliefs are maintained interpersonally through perceptions about social class, hierarchy, and nuanced judgment about perceived life chances, opportunities, and prospects (Choi, 2018). These cultural wounds and biases can carry considerable shame. Shame seems to be a ceaseless experience deeply ingrained in one's sense of self and related to less privileged social class affiliation; perhaps a price paid for membership (Russell, 1996). Individuals may find themselves distanced from their roots, which in turn distances them from themselves. This can unconsciously play out in a group, given the complexity of the class culture-bound experiences of the members and the leader. There is also a considerable interface with race and other identities, further complicating the issue. As group leaders who operate in a role of professional power, there is inadvertent maintenance of this privilege. The nature of the office setting in which providers work, the clothes they wear, the credentials on the wall and so on, can create assumptions for clients. A paradigm shift needs to occur to bring the invisible social identity of classism into the room, out of the denial, oversimplification, and minimization, to highlight members' diverse cultural histories. Without acknowledgment, there can be no equity or inclusion. Those become illusions.

The Therapy Group

Therapy groups begin with the creation of a literal and figurative agreement between the group leader and the participants. The initial session gives all participants an opportunity to assess the circumstances, monitor the environment for safety, and decide whether they are prepared to embark on the agreed-upon journey. The need to establish oneself as an individual, simultaneously becoming part of a whole, creates considerable uncertainty and anxiety. Survival and attachment are the primary tasks. The establishment of commonalities, minimizing differences, and idealizing the therapist sets the stage for an undifferentiated sort of bonding which helps members cope with their anxiety, as well as for later differentiation (Rice, 1992). On this primal level of survival, the invisible 'ism' of class can work unconsciously to help a group establish this foundation of likeness, a wish to be accepted. Suppressing classism could be a more pressing 'need' when other visible differences are present in the room. The group needs to find a non-threatening basis for coming together to confront the task of organizing themselves into a functional group (Beck & Dugo et al., 1996). Immediately the issues of developing group norms and establishing identity are prominent.

Once the group creates this initial bond, the decision to move forward begins to work towards forging a group identity which can create its own anxieties. Systems open and close boundaries. The organization of systems works to integrate and sustain members for survival, as long as the differences are not too great. Systems tend to close to differences when the groups' ability to tolerate the difference becomes too great (Agazarian, 1992). What style of communication is acceptable, competitive or cooperative, authoritarian or democratic? This exploration often begins to highlight differences in members, simultaneously working to cooperate with one another and the leader. Members assume different leadership roles which can reflect their internalized sense of self and other. Group roles may be 'thrust' upon members creating tensions within the members and the collective. This is part of the struggle for autonomy, for visibility by members as their fuller selves, not part of external or internalized projections. The tensions can become palpable, and the need to stay connected in the face of differences challenges us. Given that classism is essentially invisible, the unconscious forces will likely continue to keep those differences at bay.

Case Example: Clinical Case Vignette #1

There are three exchanges from one group experience. Each exchange describes particular group tasks that are important to understand from a leadership perspective. This first exchange illustrates the initial primary group task "survival and attachment".

First Exchange

An experiential training group, specifically for experienced mental health professionals, gathers for the first time. The leader is an older, Euro-American, cisgender woman. The membership is diverse in terms of gender, ethnicity, age, mental health disciplines as well as years of experience in the field. Members are expectedly anxious, and increasingly uncertain as the group membership is diverse, including several inexperienced participants. Before the group even begins, a conflict around membership is present. The inexperienced members worry about whether they can 'stay,' and the experienced participants question the decision-making on the part of the planning organization. The visible differences in membership involve race, gender, and age. The invisible and initially unspoken potential differences and similarities are present related to class. The group eventually bonds around the possibility that they are all 'misfits' in some way, the leftovers that were not able to be in other groups.

As groups work to forge a solid identity and establish group norms, differences between members become more apparent. This can be thought of as the 'structure and protest phase' (Rice, 1992). This is a transitional period in the time of a group, where the unconscious issues in the first phase are increasingly evident. Members begin to experience greater differences, and conflicts are emerging. As expressions of discontent in the group increase, the competence of the leader and the value of the group as a whole are at the forefront. The sense of group singularity is gone. Members become more guarded, subgroups often develop, individuals and/or subgroups can behave as if there is an enemy against whom one must defend, and the leader can be directly challenged as the anxiety around the leader's inability to protect the group from conflict and the hope for the idealized experience waivers. This is a time in the life of the group when cohesion, interpersonal mistrust, and individual psychological disorganization can be heightened. It is a time of increasing polarization. The predominant mode of interaction is competitive. The salient issues become the criteria for 'membership/belonging' and whether the group is capable of establishing a cooperative mode of interacting to solve emerging problems. It is without question the juncture at which a scapegoat can emerge as a 'solution' to the problem. The need for the group leader to be active and engaged is high. At times when group conflict is heightened it can be most effective to use group-as-a-whole interventions to help members begin to experience their commonalities and rebuild cohesion. The efforts can shift out of a competitive mode to a group where the polarities can be dissolved. It could be useful to vocalize the differences in the room including class differences that had begun to emerge. Given the visible differences age, race, gender there were many 'threats' to a sense of membership and/or belonging. Acknowledging these might have been useful in the face of the increasing polarization. This second exchange exemplifies the increasingly acknowledged conflicts in the room.

Second Exchange

Persistent themes around the therapist's competence or desirability were prominent given the group identity as a collection of 'misfits' or 'leftovers.' The group struggled with this issue of inclusion, specifically who has the right to be there, to speak. A strong subgroup emerged consisting of three senior members, two cisgender white men and one cisgender white woman. The two men and one woman were the most vocally active. The term 'power pair'' (hierarchical structure) got introduced by one of the men and became a way to describe their subgroup, although both disavowed wanting to be viewed that way. Although potential factors associated with classism (e.g., income, professional status) could be related to the formation of this subgroup of senior members, as is common in groups, these dimensions were not explicitly mentioned.

The exclusion of the vocal woman became identified. Additionally, a subgroup developed between the three trainees, more by default identification than one they necessarily would have chosen. The members who were not immediately part of a subgroup occasionally would speak but primarily identified themselves as 'outside of any conforming parameters'. The alignment within the 'power pair'' was established. This allowed the group to reveal a bit more about the experience of being 'othered,' whether as characteristic representatives of the status quo or the still-in-training, first-generation professionals. The women began having stronger voices and, at times, would protest the male paradigm that had been created around 'who is at the top of the power pair.'

The younger members were more inhibited and cautious, seeming well aware of their tenuous state of membership. The most inhibited and quiet of the younger members became a particular focus of the group. There was criticism of his unwillingness to share much and his over-intellectualization. He was the most protected by another member of this subgroup. There was considerable anxiety around inclusion, whether he could 'hold up' to the 'standards of expression' in the group. The leader needed to take a very active role in addressing the group split as well as focusing on the target of attack and helping him become more visible to the other group members. The member who had 'come to his rescue' was able to relinquish this role and return to his struggles with self-expression.

To shift from this difficult juncture in the group's life a process of reparation and integration needs to transpire (Rice, 1992). Members begin to be able to turn their awareness from one of attack to an increased awareness of their own thoughts, feelings, and impulses. The recognition of individual differences, their unique problems, and utilization of these differences become valued contributions to the group. This group stage focuses heavily on cooperation and increased interest in others. The group members slowly take more responsibility for the group and the designated leader is able to step back from a more active role. Humor and creativity enter group life. Stability and cohesion in group systems transpire as a result of integrating these differences. Systemic change reverberates through this acknowledgment and integration. Systems are energy-organizing and can be self-correcting (Agazarian, 1992). Members' ability to value one another and not fear or idealize the leader creates the basis for a new kind of commitment. The designated leader can be integrated into the group as a person while retaining the role. This third exchange describes what transpired at this most difficult time in the group, as well as the groups' desire to work together and become a whole.

Third Exchange

The group tensions increased as the conflicts around white male dominance, hierarchical power, and disavowed roles increased. Members made concerted efforts to address the issues, and to find their voices through the patterns that persisted. The more vocal members increased their attention on the quieter members. Members demonstrated more curiosity about each other's experiences without judgment or defensiveness. The increased capacity of each member and the group as a whole to tolerate the differences, and the conflicts, grew. The intimacy increased around struggles with sexuality and changing relationships contributed to the deconstruction of the barriers that had been contributing to the degrees of isolation each person felt. The subgroups vanished. There were expressions of tenderness and closeness as the time to end the experience approached. There was a freedom for the members in the deconstruction of the hierarchy/classism that was an integral part of the initial paradigm that brought the group together.

Case Discussion

The role of the designated leader shifts as the group moves through different stages. Interventions vacillate between group-as-a-whole and individual. In addition to the leader beginning the group session with the expectations for participation, this is a time to refer to the differences that are visible and invisible in the room. The group experience is an opportunity to move towards deeper understanding of self, other, and the collective.

This particular group presented difficulties around affiliation from the onset, beginning with the conflict around membership. This contributed to the difficulty the group had with an initial attachment and the sense that this would be a survivable experience. Leaders need to be more active initially in group development, particularly when conflicts are high. The leader needs to establish and maintain a sense of composure and hopefulness in the face of the conflicts (Tuttman, 1992). The issues of classism perhaps became even more invisible at first, given the overt degree of conflict around membership differences that were starkly present. The leader worked to create a therapeutic environment in which the members could explore their likenesses and sense of 'other.' The groups' emerging identity as misfits led by a rejected leader was fraught with what were likely cultural wounds, biases, loss, grief, and shame. The themes of injustices emerged as this hierarchical structure in the group developed. It particularly highlighted the ways class status is often defined by the relationship with white educated men, rather than a more direct discussion of class status. A more focused examination of what contributed to power in this group along with the leader's attunement to class status may have offered a deeper understanding of the class dynamics of this group. The jocular rivalry between the two identified 'power pair' persisted as a point of reference for the group. It became a subgroup with closed access. This groups' questions about the cisgender female leaders 'power status" were directly and indirectly addressed. This played into an ongoing less than conscious question about the leaders' competence as well as possible collusion with the status quo. All of this unconsciously supported the institutional structure and traditions, in spite of the verbal renunciations by the appointed 'power pair.'

To help the group find points of likeness as a means to create a therapeutic environment, the leader used group-as-a-whole interpretations whenever possible. Additionally, the leader would actively make bridging efforts in order to strengthen the emotional bonds between the dominant and more reticent members (Ormont, 1990). During the time in the group when the conflicts escalated, including the questioning of the therapist's neutrality, the fears of whether this experience was survivable were palpable. The leader took a very active role in intervening in the intensity of the subgrouping and developing attacks on the most differentiated member. It is important for the leader to actively maintain an empathic connection to the most differentiated member who is spotlighted at this time, as well as connecting with the other members to shift the group from this active mode of exclusion to one of self-reflection and understanding. In this process, the possibility of maximizing the group's awareness around common concerns and shared resistance, such as loss, grief, shame, and cultural wounds sets the stage for deepened understanding and connection. In this case example, the group experienced a palpable absence of tensions, increased compassion and empathy for each member, a strong sense of the collective, and the wish to continue beyond the end of the group agreement.

Clinical Case Vignette #2: Group Psychotherapy Training

Marla (they/them), a group psychotherapy trainee, is co-leading a therapy group with their group psychotherapy supervisor, Allan (he/him). This group is in a community mental health center with clients who are predominantly of low socioeconomic status and mixed racial, gender, and sexual identities.

During one of their group sessions, the group members spend much of the time discussing difficulties relating to their psychiatrists and other individual treatment team members. Members focus on the ways in which their treatment team members don't understand their struggles, and how implementing certain changes recommended by their teams is experienced as insurmountable, owing to economic and social pressures outside of their control. Multiple members note how irritating it can be when they are told to eat a more nutritious diet when their income and government benefits are often insufficient to buy expensive food that will take time to prepare. The group as a whole expresses frustration directed towards their individual treating clinicians, although no direct comments are made toward the group leaders.

Neither Marla nor Allan brings up their own identities as members of the treatment team, instead focusing on helping members share different ways they have addressed treatment recommendations they do not feel equipped to manage with their individual clinicians. Marla considers broaching the topic of relating to people across different SES backgrounds but is unsure if this would be appropriate or how to introduce the topic. Marla grew up in a low-SES household and worries that they would overly disclose or identify with group members. Marla has not told Allan about how they share similar experiences with their group members.

Debriefing

Marla and Allan debrief the group immediately following the session.

"What did you think of the exchange about the group members and their treatment teams?" Allan asks.

"I wasn't sure what to do about it, honestly," says Marla. "I realized at some point that they might have been frustrated with us, too, not just their individual clinicians."

"I found that challenging as well, and I probably could handle that better in the future," Allan nods in agreement. "They make such good points, though, don't they? It can be so difficult to imagine what it's like living on assistance, and many of them are single parents with multiple jobs. They're all trying so hard. We have no idea what it must be like."

Marla pauses, then replies, "Uh, yeah, you're right. It's hard to imagine."

Case Discussion

In this example, the supervisor has made a comment presuming the class status of their supervisee. The supervisee, in turn, experiences a sense of "othering," in which it is made clear that their identity as a therapist from a disadvantaged background is invisible in the room and perhaps should be ignored or hidden in a professional setting. This commentary silences further exploration of the experience of the therapist from a disadvantaged class background, and further, diverts away from what could be a useful discussion about class-related transference experiences for the group members. The supervisee, who may have countertransference issues around class which would be relevant to their professional development, is cornered into either flagging their otherness with their supervisor or remaining invisible. In the absence of establishing a safe environment to describe their experiences, this avenue of exploration is diverted.

When communicating with trainees, it is important to avoid assumptions about a person's background based on their appearance, manner, or academic achievements (Warnock & Hurst, 2016). Invisible identities including gender identity, sexual orientation, disability status, and class history, may be presumed in a dominant culture of middle-to-upper class, cisgender, heterosexual individuals who do not experience disability. The use of assumptive language as it refers to a person's identity reinforces implicit biases and dominant power structures, further alienating individuals with marginalized identities from professional and academic spheres (Mollett & Lackman, 2019). Rather than using assumptive language and commentary, a mentor can create a more open environment that includes discussion on topics of identity by using neutral language and inviting the trainee to share their experiences where it is safe and appropriate to do so. Questions like "What did their discussion about money bring up for you?" or "Our group members experience a great deal of adversity. I wonder what was going on for you when they were talking about that?" could offer the trainee the opportunity to describe their experiences, if those experiences feel relevant and safe to disclose. The supervisor may also be able to relate through transparent observation on how it can be difficult to address issues of class and income, leaving space for the trainee to reflect on their own experiences. In general, curiosity about a trainee's reflections on issues closely related to class identity is more useful than overly identifying with (and in this case, misidentifying with) what is presumed to be the trainee's class history.

Ethical Considerations

It is important to emphasize the ways in which power and privilege may be present in a relationship on a less-than-conscious level, particularly for the person in a greater position of power. It is important that all therapists, who are inherently inhabiting a position of power in the "therapist/client" dynamic, be aware of the impact that their power has in a group setting. The examination of any bias, including class bias, should not be seen as a competency to be "obtained" but as an ongoing process of self-reflection and education which may be challenged and changed over time (Beagan, 2018). Proceeding into relationships with clients with the belief that cultural/class competency is a singly obtainable experience leads only to perpetuate power structures through inflexibility and inability to adapt to new information as cultures change over time. On a professional level, it is important that our institutions and organizations take into account both SES and SSS when considering the class status and diversity of trainees and take care to be inclusive in our language around trainees who may be of differing class backgrounds.

Although discussion of class attitudes and identity may be a therapeutically rich topic in group, it should be made clear to therapists and group members that disclosure of marginalized, invisible identities should never be compelled or seen as required. Required or pressured disclosures of marginalized identities further reinforces power dynamics where those in a position of relative privilege may behave as if they are "entitled" to such information. Individuals of marginalized identities should not be seen as a source of education for either the group or the therapist, and it is important that therapists be mindful to avoid placing additional burdens on marginalized people to do the emotional and cognitive "work" for those of relatively greater privilege.

Attention to boundaries around identity disclosure is equally important in a mentor-mentee relationship, where boundaries around the personal and professional may feel more permeable than might be appropriate at any given time. As noted in the discussion of the therapy training vignette earlier in this chapter, a mentor or supervisor can support an environment of acceptance and safety through use of non-assumptive language and curiosity, however, this should be balanced with willingness to honor the boundaries of the trainee around their identity.

Implications for Training and Practice

Classism, like other forms of bias and systemic oppression of marginalized identities, bears special consideration in the group therapy setting and in the training of group therapy clinicians. Leaders and mentors in group psychotherapy should be encouraged to reflect on their own class identity and assumptions, and actively attend to class-related transference and countertransference dynamics within the group therapy space. Classist conflicts and disadvantages often intersect with other marginalized identities, including disability status, gender identity, sexual orientation, and race, further heightening the importance of learning to identify classist attitudes and ways in which classism may impact a person's experience of the other facets of their identity. The challenges related to class bias may be related to accurate assumptions about a person's class background, however, inaccurate assumptions (such as assuming a therapist's family of origin was middle-class or wealthy) may be just as alienating as a more "negative" stereotype.

It is of paramount importance that group psychotherapists foster environments that are accepting of varied class-related experiences. Therapists should endeavor to utilize language that encourages individuals to explore their own identities and avoid assumptive language or pronunciations about a group member's identity and be open to feedback when they have made an assumption in error. This open exchange should always be in service of the client or group as a whole, rather than for the good of the therapist themselves. There may be an unhelpful drive on the part of the therapist to "learn from" people with experiences vastly different than their own, placing undue stress and expectations on clients or trainees from less-advantaged class status to "help" the therapist in a position of power. This pressure to provide information, which may not be useful to the group or the individual clients in question, can be experienced as voyeuristic and reinforces the felt experience of being "othered." Therapists have an ethical duty to reflect and educate themselves on class bias, while simultaneously providing space for people of differently advantaged class status to describe their experience without undue projections and expectations.

Examination of classist dynamics affecting therapists, including therapists from disadvantaged backgrounds in the professional space, is crucial to the development of skills to address transferential class-related dilemmas in group psychotherapy. Group therapy as a profession has much work to do in supporting the training of therapists from a wider variety of class backgrounds. Further research and literature on these complicated topics are necessary as the field continues to explore the nature of identity and the importance of interpersonal power dynamics in the group therapy space.

References

Association of American Medical Colleges. (2008, January). *Diversity of U.S. medical students by parental income*. www.census.gov/hhes/www/income/histinc/h01ar.html.

Agazarian, Y. (1992). Contemporary theories of group psychotherapy: A systems approach to the group-as-a-whole. *International Journal of Group Psychotherapy, 42*(2), 177–203. https://doi.org/10.1080/00207284.1992.11490685.

American Psychological Association. (2002). *Socioeconomic status discrimination due to sexual orientation and gender identity*. www.apa.org/pi.

Ballinger, L. & Wright, J. (2007). 'Does class count?' Social class and counselling. *Counselling and Psychotherapy Research, 7*(3), 157–163. https://doi.org/10.1080/14733140701571316.

Beagan, B. L. (2018). A critique of cultural competence: Assumptions, limitations, and alternatives. In: Frisby, C. & O'Donohue, W. (Eds), *Cultural competence in applied psychology*. Cham: Springer. https://doi.org/10.1007/978-3-319-78997-2_6.

Beck, A. P. (1981). A study of group phase development and emergent leadership. *Group, 5*(4), 48–54. www.jstor.org/stable/41718048.

Choi, N.-Y. & Miller, M. J. (2018). Social class, classism, stigma, and college students' attitudes toward counseling. *The Counseling Psychologist, 46*(6), 761–785. https://doi.org/10.1177/001100001879.

Christophers, B. & Marr, M. C. (2022). Pendergrast, T. R. Medical school admission policies disadvantage low-Income applicants. The *Permanente Journal, 26*(2), 172–176. https://doi.org/10.7812/TPP/21.18.

Cook, J. M. & Lawson, G. (2016). Counselors' social class and socioeconomic status understanding and awareness. *Journal of Counseling and Development, 94*(4), 442–453. https://doi.org/10.1002/jcad.12103.

Cook, J. M. (2019). *Add-Wellness*: A humanistic model to conceptualize addiction. *College of Education Faculty Research and Publications, 539*, 46–47. https://epublications.marquette.edu/edu_fac/539

Cook, J. M. & O'Hara, C. C. (2020). An emerging theory of the persistence of social class microaggressions: an interpretative phenomenological study. *Counselling Psychology Quarterly, 33*(4), 516–540. https://doi.org/10.1080/09515070.2019.1596880.

Demakakos, P., Nazroo, J., Breeze, E., & Marmot, M. (2008). Socioeconomic status and health: the role of subjective social status. *Social Science Medicine, 67*(2), 330–340. https://doi.org/10.1016/j.socscimed.2008.03.038.

Dougall, J. L. & Schwartz, R. C. (2011). The influence of client socioeconomic status on psychotherapists' attributional biases and countertransference reaction. *American Journal of Psychotherapy, 65*(3), 249–265. https://doi.org/10.1176/APPI.PSYCHOTHERAPY.2011.65.3.249.

Gelso, C. J. & Mohr, J. J. (2001). The working alliance and the transference/countertransference relationship: Their manifestation with racial/ ethnic and sexual orientation minority clients and therapists. *Applied & Preventative Psychology, 10*(1), 51–68. https://doi.org/10.1016/S0962-1849(05)80032-0.

Klein, R. H., Bernard, H. S., & Singer, D. L. (1992). *Handbook of contemporary group psychotherapy: Contributions from object relations, self-psychology, and social systems theories*. International Universities Press, Inc.

Kim, S. & Cardemil, E. (2012). Effective psychotherapy with low-income clients: The importance of attending to social class. *Journal of Contemporary Psychotherapy, 42*(1), 27–35. https://doi.org/10.1007/s10879-011-9194-0.

Lavell, E. F. (2014). Beyond charity: Social class and classism in counselling. *Canadian Journal of Counselling and Psychotherapy, 48*(3). https://cjc-rcc.ucalgary.ca/article/view/60986.

Lott, B. (2012). The social psychology of class and classism. *American Psychologist, 67*(8), 650.

McDowell, T., Brown, A. L., Cullen, N., & Duyn, A. (2013). Social class in family therapy education: Experiences of low SES students. *Journal of Marital and Family Therapy, 39*(1), 72–86. https://doi.org/10.1111/j.1752-0606.2011.00281.x.

McEvoy, C., Clarke, V., & Thomas, Z. (2021). 'Rarely discussed but always present': Exploring therapists' accounts of the relationship between social class, mental health, and therapy. *Counselling & Psychotherapy Research, 21*(2), 324–334. https://doi.org/10.1002/capr.12382.

Mollet, A. L. & Lackman, B. (2019). Asexual student invisibility and erasure in higher education. In *Rethinking LGBTQIA students and collegiate contexts: Identity, policies, and campus climate*, 78–98. https://doi.org/10.4324/9780429447297.

National Center for Education Statistics. (2015). Postsecondary attainment: Differences by socioeconomic status. In *The Condition of Education*. https://nces.ed.gov/programs/coe/pdf/coe_tva.pdf.

Newton, K. (2010) A two-fold unveiling: Unmasking classism in group work. *The Journal for Specialists in Group Work, 35*(3), 212–219. https://doi.org/10.1080/01933922.2010.492906.

Ormont, L. (1990). The craft of bridging. *International Journal of Group Psychotherapy, 40*(1), 3–17. https://doi.org/10.1080/00207284.1990.11490580.

Rice, M. E., Harris, G. T., & Cormier, C. A. (1992). An evaluation of a maximum security therapeutic community for psychopaths and other mentally disordered offenders. *Law and Human Behavior, 16*(4), 399–412. https://doi.org/10.1007/BF02352266.

Russell, G. (1996) Internalized classism. *Women & Therapy, 18*(3–4), 59–71. https://doi.org/10.1300/J015v18n03_07,

Shapiro, T. M., Meschede, T., & Osoro, S. (2013, February). The roots of the widening racial wealth gap: Explaining the black-white economic divide. *Institute on Assets and Social Policy: Research and Policy Brief*, 1–8.

Smith, L. (2005). Psychotherapy, classism, and the poor: Conspicuous by their absence. *American Psychologist, 60*(7), 687. https://doi.org/10.1037/0003-066X.60.7.687.

Smith, L. (2008). Positioning classism within counseling psychology's social justice agenda. *The Counseling Psychologist, 36*(6), 895–924. https://doi.org/10.1177/0011000007309861.

Smith, L., Foley, P. F., & Chaney, M. P. (2008). Addressing classism, ableism, and heterosexism in counselor education. *Journal of Counseling & Development, 86*(3), 303–309. https://doi.org/10.1002/j.1556-6678.2008.tb00513.x

Sue, D. W., Sue, D., Neville, H. A., & Smith, L. (2012). *Counseling the culturally diverse: Theory and practice*. John Wiley & Sons, Inc.

Taylor, D. M. (2018). Americans with disabilities: 2014. *US Census Bureau*, 1–32. www.census.gov/content/dam/Census/library/publications/2018/demo/p70-152.pdf.

Thompson, M. N., Cole, O. D., & Nitzarim, R. S. (2012). Recognizing social class in the psychotherapy relationship: A grounded theory exploration of low-income clients. *Journal of counseling psychology, 59*(2), 208. https://doi.org/10.1037/a0027534.

Titus, M. A. (2006). Understanding college degree completion of students with low socioeconomic status: The influence of the institutional financial context. In *Research in Higher Education, 47*(4), 371–398. https://doi.org/10.1007/s11162-005-9000-5.

Tuttman, S. (1992). The role of the therapist from an object relations perspective. In R. H. Klein, H. S. Bernard, & D. S. Singer (Eds), *Handbook of contemporary group psychotherapy* (pp. 241–278). International Universities Press.

Warnock, D. M. & Hurst, A. L. (2016). "The poor kids' table": Organizing around an invisible and stigmatized identity in flux. *Journal of Diversity in Higher Education, 9*(3), 261–276. https://doi.org/10.1037/dhe0000029.

Wiley, J. & Manstead, A. S. R. (2018). The psychology of social class: How socioeconomic status impacts thought, feelings, and behavior. *British Journal of Social Psychology, 57*(2), 267–291. https://doi.org/10.1111/bjso.12251.

Yan, Y. & Gai, X. (2022). High achievers from low family socioeconomic status families: Protective factors for academically resilient students. *International Journal of Environmental Research Public Health, 19*(23), 15882. https://doi.org/10.3390/ijerph192315882.

5 An Unsacred Silence

Conceptualizing Religious Dynamics in Group Psychotherapy

Mendel Horowitz and Avidan Milevsky

Cultural competency is an essential component of general medical care (Betancourt et al., 2003) and, in particular, psychotherapy (American Psychological Association, 2003). According to the Pew Forum on Religion and Public Life (2019) over 90 percent of Americans report a belief in a universal power or God and more than half indicate that religion is an essential element of their life. The importance of religion in the lives of individuals can also be seen in the growing body of literature attending to issues of religion, spirituality, and well-being (Damianakis et al., 2018; Milevsky & Eisenberg, 2012; Pargament, 2007; Walker et al., 2012a; Walker et al., 2012b; Wilchek & Aviad, 2014).

Conceptual Framework

Several attempts have been made to differentiate between the construct of religion and spirituality (Hill et al., 2000). Although overlaps between the two concepts exist, generally, religion is seen as the set of cognitions, emotions, behaviors, and experiences that emanate from a quest and contact with a higher sanctified entity occurring within a structured religious institution. On the other hand, spirituality is accepted to be experienced on a more personal level and via independent exploration and practice (Abernethy et al., 2019).

The concept of religion as a "six-dimensional organism" is described by Smart (1969) and reviewed by Rennie (1999). In this conception, the religious experience can be organized as 1) ritual; 2) mythological; 3) doctrinal; 4) ethical; 5) social; and 6) experiential. In his review of Smart (1969), Rennie (1999) describes the following six dimensions of religious experience: 1) *Ritual* refers to outer behaviors coordinated "with an inner intention to make contact with, or to participate in, the invisible world." 2) *Mythological* refers to stories about God and historical events of religious significance in a tradition through which the invisible world is symbolized. 3) *Doctrinal* refers to the "attempt to give system, clarity, and intellectual power to what is revealed through the mythological and symbolic language of religious faith and ritual." 4) *Ethical* is the codes of belief and behavior that govern personal conduct and communal interactions. 5) *Social* norms are how religion is institutionalized through teachings and expectations. Finally, 6) *Experiential* refers to the personal encounter with an invisible world that is beyond ritual and social interaction.

Group psychotherapy can be seen as a spiritual community where group members work to identify, integrate, and transform aspects of themselves and their relationships with one another (Jebreel et al., 2018). Group therapy and spirituality share several features which, when combined, can create a potent milieu. For example, both group work and spirituality contain themes of hope, universality, and altruism, making for a natural integration of both. Furthermore, according to Jacques (1998) "religious and spiritual themes, when carefully

DOI: 10.4324/9781003455783-7

and thoughtfully explored, reveal rich data concerning group members' intrapsychic conflicts, their interpersonal relationships, and their sense of self." While non-religious clients might come to group treatment with existential dilemmas as well as interpersonal conflicts, religious clients can have particular spiritual or religious conflicts from their past that manifest during group interactions. Considering the multidimensional nature of, and the interplay between, group psychotherapy and the religious experience, group resistances and transferences can manifest differently in relation to each of the six dimensions of religion as will be reviewed in the upcoming case example.

The Six Dimensions of Religious Experience in Family-Centered Faith Communities

In the United States, research indicates that religion is a significant factor in family relationships (Mahoney et al., 2001). Among religions, Christianity, Judaism, Mormonism, and Islam are all monotheistic, trace their roots to Abraham and his covenants, and are explicitly family-centered (Agius & Chircop, 1998; Marks & Dollahite, 2001). When religious Christian, Jewish, Mormon, and Muslim parents were interviewed regarding the importance of religious family interactions, rituals, and practices in their families, Marks (2004) reports the importance of teaching by example or "behavior-belief congruence" as central to the family constellation. Parents who confine religious practice or observance to particular circumstances or display behaviors incongruous with their beliefs dilute the significance of religious faith for their children and often experience associated regret.

In religious families whose members strive together to fulfill spiritual goals or sacred purposes, an amalgam of practices, beliefs, and expectations can contribute to stability and shared purpose. Examples of family-centered religious behaviors include a Jewish father blessing a cup of wine for his family on Friday evening in honor of the Sabbath, a Muslim family observing Ramadan to honor Allah, a Mormon family holding Family Home Evening each Monday night, and an Episcopalian family singing grace each evening at dinner (Dollahite & Marks, 2005).

While religious observance can offer its adherents a sense of fulfillment, harmony, and satisfaction, the effects of noncompliance can be devastating. When religious clients enter group therapy, their feelings of shame and remorse can become a barrier to dialogue and a clinician who is not attuned can unwittingly collude with a client's defensive reactions (Cornish et al., 2014). The multiculturally competent clinician will seek to understand clients' theories of problems, change, and health as they relate to presenting concerns (Arredondo et al., 1996).

Group Interventions

The focus on integrating religion and spirituality in psychotherapy has primarily revolved around its value in individual psychotherapy. The integration of both religion and spirituality in psychotherapy is particularly poignant, considering that studies indicate that clients regard issues of religion and spirituality as an integral part of their turmoil and recovery (Pargament, 2007; Shafranske, 2013). Furthermore, the majority of clients in a US-based study reported a desire to discuss matters of religion and spirituality in a session (Rose et al., 2001). Most importantly, the incorporation of religious and spiritual themes within the psychotherapeutic milieu has been shown to have a positive impact on therapeutic outcomes (Pargament, 2007).

The literature on religion, spirituality, and psychotherapy has largely ignored its utility in group psychotherapy (Cornish & Wade, 2010; Post et al., 2013). This oversight may be driven by a broader uneasiness in discussing matters of religion publicly (Cornish et al., 2013; Richards & Potts, 1995). Others have attributed this neglect to a lack of training in the identification of religious and spiritual themes in group dynamics (Post et al., 2013; Young et al., 2002).

The inattention to religious and spiritual issues in group psychotherapy is an oversight. First, more broadly, group therapy has been shown to create positive change by helping group members learn new ways to think of themselves and others as well as evaluate and adapt what feels congruent to their lives in relation to others (Bartkowski, 2000; Karp, 1992; Mason-Schrock, 1996; Truax, 2002). Within the group setting, the distressed individual can feel less stigmatized and isolated and more capable of handling concerns as a result of group members' guidance and feedback about the shared problem (Humphreys, 2004). This mutual assistance can enhance members' self-esteem and shape their self-identity (Levine, et al., 2005).

Spirituality and religion may offer hope, encourage altruism, and provide perspective and meaning in the face of existential challenges. Considering these strengths to group psychotherapy, the active or passive apprehension toward addressing topics of religion and spirituality in group psychotherapy is particularly unfortunate considering the benefits of such incorporation on group psychotherapeutic processes and outcomes (Cornish et al., 2013; Wade et al., 2014). Issues of religion and spirituality may be particularly relevant in interpersonal process groups. Among the various forms of therapeutic groups, interpersonal process groups are most dependent on group cohesion (Yalom & Leszcz, 2020). Forsyth (2010) indicates that an essential element of a group is found in the relationships connecting members. Furthermore, in groups that emphasize member interaction, a positive relationship between cohesion and outcome exists (Burlingame et al., 2013).

Owing to the difficult nature of public discussions about religion, engaging in conversations about matters of faith in group psychotherapy, although challenging, can set the stage for open and honest dialog about uncomfortable subject matter. In fact, Yarhouse and Beckstead (2011) found the group milieu particularly transformative in discussing difficult subject matter such as sexual topics and religious tensions. Despite the potential benefits of this exploration, Horowitz and Milevsky (2020) have shown that the possibility of collective resistance and transference may be heightened when working with group members whose religious experience encompasses multidimensional concerns. Hence, to address religious dynamics in group psychotherapy effectively an understanding of religious-specific resistance and transference is essential.

Group Resistances and Transferences

Although group therapy is an effective and widely utilized form of psychotherapy that provides individuals with an opportunity to address their mental health concerns in a supportive group setting, like any therapeutic process, group therapy can be influenced by various dynamics, including resistance and transference (Billow, 2006). Resistance refers to the unconscious defense mechanisms employed by individuals to avoid confronting painful emotions or engaging in therapeutic change (Hagedorn, 2011). In group therapy, resistance can manifest in several ways. Some participants may be reluctant to share personal experiences or emotions, fearing judgment or vulnerability. Others may engage in disruptive behaviors, such as dominating discussions or withdrawing from participation. Understanding the underlying causes of resistance is crucial for therapists to create a safe and supportive environment that encourages participants to explore their resistance and process it constructively.

Transference occurs when individuals unconsciously transfer emotions, desires, and expectations from past significant events or relationships onto the group members or the therapist. In group therapy, participants may project their unresolved feelings onto their peers or perceive the therapist as a figure from their past. These transference dynamics can profoundly impact the therapeutic process by influencing group dynamics, forming alliances, or hindering progress. Skillful facilitation and the therapeutic alliance formed between the therapist and the group members are essential in recognizing and addressing transference issues to promote progress and growth.

Resistance and transference are interconnected phenomena in group therapy (Billow, 2001). Resistance often arises as a defense mechanism against the vulnerability and potential emotional exposure associated with transference. Participants may resist opening up or exploring certain topics, owing to fear of repeating past negative experiences or the discomfort of facing unresolved conflicts. Recognizing and understanding these dynamics can provide therapists with valuable insights into the group members' internal struggles and enable them to tailor interventions that facilitate growth and positive change. Managing resistance and transference in group therapy requires a delicate balance between creating a safe space for exploration and challenging participants to confront their underlying issues. Therapists must foster trust, empathy, and open communication to encourage participants to express their resistance and explore transference dynamics openly. By doing so, group members can gain insight into their emotional patterns, develop healthier coping strategies, and establish more authentic connections with others. Recognizing various "dimensions" of religious experience can enable a clinician to better identify and resolve religious-based resistance and transference conflicts that arise in group interactions.

Religious and Spiritual Competencies for the Religious Client

Although significant contributions have been made in considering racial and ethnic identity, the examination of religion and spirituality as integral components of personal identity in psychotherapeutic treatment has received less attention. The intersection between religious and spiritual identities with race, ethnicity, and other cultural identities has been addressed even less. As a result, limited training is available in applying clinical practice that acknowledges and integrates issues of religion and spirituality in client's life-perspectives, individuality, and mental health (Pearce et al., 2019; Sue, et al., 2009). A sensitive inquiry into the religious and spiritual needs and orientations of clients can enhance psychiatric assessment and taking appropriate action based on the elicited information can facilitate recovery and healing during treatment (Whitley & Jarvis, 2015 & 2012). Rassool (2015) stresses the imperative to develop a better understanding of the mental health needs and concerns of the Muslim community, and Gabbay and colleagues (2017) insist the successful treatment of Orthodox Jews in psychotherapy depends on the management of deeply held spiritual beliefs, a complex code of ritual observance, a balance between client autonomy and rabbinic authority, and fear of the stigma associated with mental illness and other issues.

Considering these features of Orthodox Judaism, an analysis of group psychotherapy with Orthodox Jews is particularly valuable in understanding the process and content of integrating religion and spirituality in group work. While the category "Orthodox Jews" is difficult to define because of variations in the meaning of the term (Wikler, 1986), the breadth and intensity of Orthodox Jewish observance result in numerous peculiarities, idiosyncrasies, and sensitivities (Silverstein, 1995) that make psychotherapy challenging. While the opportunity to hear other members disclose concerns similar to their own can be a powerful source of relief in group therapy (Yalom & Leszcz, 2020), group therapy can be particularly challenging for Orthodox Jewish men as the numerous peculiarities, idiosyncrasies, and sensitivities of their lifestyles can make sharing their deepest concerns intimidating (Shapiro, 1999; Silverstein, 1995).

Shame and Guilt in Orthodox Jewish Culture

Group therapy offers a unique and powerful platform for individuals to confront and address deeply rooted emotions such as shame and guilt. Shame, an intense emotional response to a perceived personal failure, arises from a profound sense of unworthiness or inadequacy (Wright, 1994). It is often accompanied by self-blame and a desire to hide or withdraw. Shame can be insidious, hindering personal growth and well-being, and thriving in isolation (Gans & Weber, 2000; Goffnett et al., 2020). Group therapy provides a safe and empathetic environment where shame can be explored and transformed collectively (Thompson & Girz, 2020).

Guilt, on the other hand, stems from a sense of responsibility for wrongdoing or harm caused to others. While guilt can serve as a moral compass, excessive or unresolved guilt can be detrimental to one's mental health. It is important that group clinicians have a working understanding of how to conceptualize religious guilt dynamics in clinical settings so that they might facilitate working with guilt in a way that is associated with positive outcomes. In a review of the relationship between religion, guilt, and mental health, Faiver and his colleagues (2000) distinguish between guilt that enhances or impedes personal growth. When failing to live up to a religious ideal, a wrongdoer might experience fear of punishment, loss of self-esteem, or feelings of isolation (Narramore, 1974). Bulka (1987) describes the relationship between guilt, low self-esteem, and collective guilt within a psychological framework and from a Judaic vantage point that emphasizes transmuting guilt toward positive expression. Group therapy offers an opportunity for individuals to share their experiences and receive feedback, helping them gain perspective and learn healthier ways of addressing guilt. By encouraging accountability without judgment, group therapy fosters personal growth and healing.

One of the key benefits of group therapy lies in the recognition and validation of shared experiences. When individuals struggling with shame and guilt realize that others have similar feelings, a sense of belonging emerges. The group becomes a supportive network where participants can express themselves authentically and find acceptance. This shared experience reduces the isolation associated with shame and guilt, creating a space for empathy, understanding, and healing.

Furthermore, in group therapy, participants have the opportunity to challenge negative self-perceptions associated with shame and guilt. Through open dialogue and feedback, individuals gain new perspectives on their actions, allowing for self-reflection and personal growth. Group members can provide support, reassurance, and encouragement, aiding in the development of healthier self-concepts and coping mechanisms.

As group members work through their shame and guilt, they develop resilience and empowerment. Witnessing the progress and growth of others in the group inspires individuals to confront their own emotional burdens. The collective support within the group fosters a sense of community, where participants learn from one another's journeys and draw strength from the transformative experiences of their peers.

Dein (2013) examines psychoanalytic, theological, and cultural theories purporting to account for the historical link between Judaism and guilt. In his celebrated code of Jewish law, Maimonides (Mishneh Torah: Chapter 1) regards verbal confession as a positive Biblical precept fulfilled by the declaration: "I implore You, God, I sinned, I transgressed, I committed iniquity before You by doing the following. Behold, I regret and am embarrassed about my deeds. I promise never to repeat this act again." Each morning, Orthodox Jewish adherents recite prayers that include the invocation "Do not bring us into the hands of sin, nor into the hands of transgression and wrongdoing, nor into the hands of trial, nor into the hands of scorn" (Scherman, 1981).

In addition to the inevitability of religious guilt, the prospect of social humiliation looms large among Orthodox Jews. Hakak (2011) sees the Orthodox community as an enclave culture that chooses to separate itself from mainstream society. Insular communities provide Orthodox Jews with cohesion and with numerous prosocial opportunities, from subsidized education and medical referrals to childcare and matchmaking. At the same time, noteworthy information and gossip travel fast in tight-knit communities, and reputations are closely guarded.

In all clinical populations, to both build a therapeutic alliance and resolve discomfort, therapists must recognize, acknowledge, and address client experiences of shame (Dearing & Tangney, 2011). While attitudes about shame and forgiveness differ among various Jewish denominations (Cohen et al., 2013), the experience of guilt and responsibility among Orthodox Jews overall in psychotherapy can be profound as they are exposed to new or previously unacknowledged feelings (Hess, 2014). In process groups of Orthodox Jewish men, the risk of empathic failure can be pronounced when one member's shameful disclosure resonates with group members and clinicians and pulls them to stay silent rather than speak explicitly about their shared experiences of shame.

Case Example and Discussion

The case example is used to describe unique aspects of integrating issues of religion and spirituality in group psychotherapy. Particular attention is given to resistances and transferences in relation to each of the six dimensions of religion together with addressing shame and guilt in the group milieu. To capture these unique elements, the case example describes the treatment of Orthodox Jews in group therapy. As noted, considering this population's deeply held spiritual beliefs, complex code of ritual observance, the balance between autonomy and rabbinic authority, and fear of the stigma associated with mental illness (Gabbay et al., 2017), a study of group dynamics with Orthodox Jews offers a fertile ground for the intricacy of addressing religious issues in psychotherapy, and particularly, issues of resistances, transferences, shame, and guilt.

The interpersonal process group was led by the first author of this chapter, a 51-year-old, American-Israeli male family therapist who self-identifies as "Orthodox" and considers himself a member of the same broad-ranging community as the Orthodox Jewish participants. The open group consisted of eight men who ranged in age from 35 to 65 years (For further description of this unique group see Horowitz and Milevsky, 2020).

While group participants displayed observable differences in style and assumed dissimilarities in ideology, each was readily identifiable as Orthodox by his head-covering, ritual fringes, and modest attire (Berman, 2000). In the style of Israeli ultra-Orthodox Jews, one group participant wore a long black formal coat and a black wide-brimmed hat. Four members wore simple sport coats and black fedoras while other members sported more contemporary styles of dress. Each participant was of Ashkenazi descent and no member was a loyal adherent of any particular sect. Each of these men immersed themselves in Jewish life and tradition and adhered strictly to kosher dietary laws, Sabbath observance, and laws of family purity which relate to sexual relations. By self-report, these men avoided popular and secular culture in degrees of flexibility, lived in self-contained communities, dedicated time each day to prayer and to studying religious texts, and recognized the authority of the Talmud and the Shulchan Aruch, the code of Jewish law that specifically guides daily practice (Cohen et al., 2013).

Core membership remained relatively intact throughout a five-year period. All participants were husbands and fathers who sought help with relationship distress and managing varying degrees of aggressiveness, loneliness, and emotional detachment. The group met weekly for 1.5 hours at a psychotherapy clinic that offers subsidized treatment for under-served religious populations in Jerusalem. Names in these accounts are fictional. Dialogue has been recreated from supervisory and case notes.

Group Development

To attract traditional men with a more welcoming framework than "interpersonal process group therapy," the group was advertised initially as a "Parenting Skills Training For Fathers." In the beginning, the group concentrated on skill-building and understanding the theoretical basis of anger and self-restraint before agreeing to engage in a more process-oriented modality. Beginning with nominally embarrassing child-rearing and relationship concerns, group participants would for a long time avoid their more shameful emotional injuries. When lessons and recommendations proved insufficient, the men understood the limited efficacy of psychoeducation. The methodology of an interpersonal process group and its virtues would become appreciated only with time. The group's shift from instructive to collaborative learning was leader-inspired and self-determined but not assigned.

Treatment Content

The relationship between shame and the six dimensions of religious experience is exemplified by an interaction that occurred during the group's fifth year. During this meeting, Baruch revealed a secret that caused him humiliation. To learn from each other how to better manage family time, Baruch and the others had been discussing their weekend routines. The Sabbath is an opportunity for spiritual and material nurturing, and the men turned to each other for advice about how to better fulfill their religious and paternal roles. As the fathers began to strategize and share their experiences, Baruch noticeably withdrew before suddenly announcing his disgrace. A father to several rambunctious sons and husband to one "intolerable" spouse, the burly man had in the past shared mostly negative impressions of them. He described his sense of being overwhelmed by his family. Until verbalizing them that evening, Baruch shouldered the weight of his failures alone. Estranged from his family and isolated from his congregation, Baruch was the group's least forthcoming member, whose detached presence placed other members on edge. "The centrality of Sabbath and its wasted potential has become an unbearable burden," disclosed Baruch, "as has my loneliness, humiliation, and regret."

Initially, Baruch's disclosure was met with utter silence. Group members appeared stunned and were rendered speechless by Baruch's vulnerability. The therapist imagined his own religious failures, and when glancing around the room, could not find appropriate words to address what they presumed to be feelings of vicarious shame. After some quiet moments, the therapist recognized the group's empathic failure and made efforts to acknowledge and address Baruch's shame. "We wonder what you heard in our silence," the therapist addressed Baruch. "When you all were silent, I felt even more guilty and ashamed," Baruch mumbled, "and I was sorry to have opened my mouth." "Talking about my family is one thing," Baruch hesitantly continued, "but admitting that I hardly observe the Sabbath is even worse."

The Six Dimensions of Religious Experience Relating to Sabbath Observance

For some Orthodox Jewish men, their identity is more clearly related to the implications of their observance than to their identity as persons. In this vignette, the shame that Baruch experienced was induced by implications from each of the six dimensions of his religious experience and recognized by the therapist, himself an Orthodox Jew. The sacredness of the Sabbath and its implications for Orthodox Jews remain unrivaled (Marks et al., 2018). Unlike space, Heschel (1951) finds time to be the "heart of existence," and the Sabbath to be the dimension of time "wherein man meets God." To Orthodox Jews, the Sabbath is more than a practical day for rest and renewal. For an Orthodox Jewish father to fulfill the Biblical command to "remember the Sabbath and keep it holy" (English Standard Version Bible, 2001) with his family, he must engage with *ritual, mythological, doctrinal, ethical, social, and experiential* elements.

Sabbath rituals include ceremonies, prayers, and the cessation of work activities. Sabbath mythologies include oral traditions and teachings about the significance of tradition. Sabbath doctrine involves biblical and rabbinic directives and a vast system of learning that imparts meaning to ritual observance. Codes of ethics govern personal conduct and communal interactions on the Sabbath. Sabbath services in a synagogue are an expected element of Orthodox observance. Most significantly, Sabbath is intended to inspire a personal encounter with an invisible world that is beyond ritual and social interaction (Bix, 2020; Frank et al., 1997; Smith-Gabai & Ludwig, 2011). For those who observe it, the Sabbath can be a precious day of joy that is eagerly awaited throughout the week and can improve feelings of mental well-being rather than a day of restrictions (Dein & Loewenthal, 2013). For Baruch to disclose his painful Sabbath experiences to a group of peers, the associated shame was immense.

As exemplified in the vignette, Sabbath observance for Orthodox Jewish men comprises rituals linked to mythological, doctrinal, ethical, social, and experiential elements of religious practice. The six dimensions of religious experience in Judaism are indistinct and tend to overlap. Lazar et al. (2002) examined the content and structure of self-reported motivation for Jewish religious behavior and identify multiple factors of impulse. Aronson et al. (2019) describe the ways in which contemporary Jews engage with their Jewish identities vary and report survey responses dealing with culture, community, nationality, and religious practices to understand Jewish engagement.

For Orthodox Jews, defining ritual as a "sequence of behaviors" is problematic. The biblical verse "Because this people draw near with their mouth and honor me with their lips, while their hearts are far from me, and their fear of me is a commandment taught by men" (English Standard Version Bible, 2001, Isa. 29:13) is understood by Rabbinic authorities as an exhortation against rote worship (Davis & Karo, 1996). Within Orthodox Jewish culture, the performance of any ritual must include elements of focused attention and inspiration to be considered worthy. The pro forma execution of religious ritual by an Orthodox Jew might include conflicting feelings of satisfaction, indifference, and even shame.

Interventions and Their Impact

In this vignette, the group was faced with a revelation of personal shame aroused, in part, by a member's failure to live up to religious and cultural expectations. The therapist recognized the challenge of staging a meaningful Sabbath because he felt at times similar about his own religious responsibilities. In ensuing conversations, other group members disclosed to Baruch that he was not alone in feeling burdened by his family and faith. After failing to react initially, the therapist initiated repair by acknowledging and addressing Baruch, and subsequently processing the group's traumatic reaction.

Being attuned to a client's shame is an important aspect of all psychotherapies, and when a therapist fails to recognize a client's shame, the client's shame-related problems will likely persist (Dearing & Tangney, 2011). In group psychotherapy, the danger of empathic failure is magnified, as clinicians find themselves swept along by group-wide emotions (Stone, 2001). When faced with Baruch's humiliation, the therapist was initially affected by the group's emotional contagion and his own religiocultural countertransference (Abernethy & Lancia, 1998). In subsequent meetings, Baruch and others would learn to offer empathic statements in place of silence when a group member disclosed feelings of shame.

Basic Strategies for Working With Orthodox Jewish Men

Numerous factors can contribute to the success of a process group. Barlow and Burlingame (2006) delineate multiple domains of effective treatment, including member and leader characteristics, small-group processes, and group structure. In addition to a leader's encouragement of beneficial group processes, group cohesion, defined as "member-to-member high positive emotional relatedness," encourages the disclosure of meaningful material and can lead to meaningful feedback among group members (Burlingame et al., 2019). In a homogeneous group of Orthodox Jewish men, while member and leader characteristics undoubtedly vary, a shared Orthodox identity among group members can contribute to group cohesion and can also present particular challenges. Similarly, a clinician from the same community might confer a feeling of safety and simultaneously raise anxieties that a clinician from another community would not arouse. In addition, the transferences of an Orthodox Jewish clinician will be different from those of a clinician who does not identify as an Orthodox Jew.

Because the scope of Orthodox Judaism encompasses religious, spiritual, and social concerns, and so dramatically affects the minutiae of how Orthodox Jews communicate and behave, an effective group clinician will need to apply a variety of competencies in comparison to an individual therapist or clinician working with a heterogeneous non-Orthodox group. In addition to cohesion, the possibility of collective resistance and transference may be heightened in a homogeneous group of Orthodox Jewish men, and a clinician will need specific skills to reveal and resolve them.

To empathize with the shame and loneliness associated with transgression against religious and cultural expectations within homogeneous groups of Orthodox Jewish men, a knowledgeable clinician will be conscious of the severity of Orthodox Judaism's ethical and social norms, and respectful of its traditions. Along with the benefits of cultural recognition, Orthodox Jewish clinicians might be affected by negative countertransferences and the need to manage personal emotional reactions. Conversely, a non-Orthodox clinician may need to make an explicit effort to experience empathy for seemingly minor religious infractions or beliefs from a non-Orthodox perspective that have significant salience for Orthodox Jews. A clinician of any persuasion will be sensitive to the possibility of collective group discomfort and demonstrate kindness by suspending judgments and acknowledging personal ambivalence and shame.

Shame and Loneliness of Nonconformity to Religious and Cultural Expectations

After committing an offense or failing to live up to a cultural expectation, individuals may feel badly about themselves, feel badly about their actions or inaction, or experience a combination of uncomfortable feelings. The shame experienced within homogeneous groups of Orthodox Jewish men may be similar to the discomfort experienced by members of other groups. Studies identify multiple defenses that may suggest the subterranean workings of shame in group therapy and conclude that "the best antidote for shame's neglect is a heightened readiness to detect it" (Gans & Weber, 2000; Goffnett et al., 2020). These defenses were evident in the therapist's experience with the workings of shame within this homogeneous group of Orthodox Jewish men. Specifically, group members focused on themes that stressed similarities among members, avoided here-and-now material, and preserved the illusion of the leader's infallibility.

A successful therapy group is one in which members can fully reveal their sense of inadequacy without experiencing the condemnation and rejection that they expect from others (Hahn, 1994; Yalom & Leszcz, 2020). Following the recommendations of Nicholas (1993), the therapist was able to address a group member's shame without being judgmental, by becoming aware of his own biases and values in the context of ongoing supervision. A sensitive clinician will invite vulnerability, suspend judgment, and encourage empathic statements instead of silence in response to a group member's disclosure of personal shame.

Ethical Considerations

Unlike when psychology distinguished itself from religion, recent researchers have recognized a commonality between religion and counseling in their capacity to effect change in people, to develop maturity and human functioning at a higher level, and to facilitate but also hinder human potential (Miller, 2003). As individuals vary in their relationships with spirituality or religion, a culturally competent clinician would appreciate these differences and engage with spiritual and religious themes accordingly during assessment and treatment. Nonreligious and religious clinicians alike would need to become aware of personal biases and recognize how the client attributes personal meanings to religion and spirituality to establish rapport. To address spiritual and religious themes effectively, it is essential for clinicians to understand spirituality and religion in the context of a broader meaning of culture and to become aware of and open to learning about beliefs and culturally related values in themselves and their clients.

Establishing cultural competency in addressing spirituality and religion in counseling and psychotherapy requires clinicians to seek appropriate training, education, consultation, and supervision. Training, including the use of role-playing and modeling, could target improvements in therapeutic skills, such as maintaining attitudes of empathy, care, acceptance, and non-judgment, as they relate to spiritual and religious concerns (Lefforge et al., 2020). Clinicians who are sensitive to clients' concerns and expectations relating to spiritual and religious concerns are more likely to create working alliances and avoid ethical violations in practice (Maximo, 2019).

Intersectionality in Culturally Homogeneous Group Treatment

According to the American Group Psychotherapy Association (2023), "intersectionality" is a term that considers the overlapping identities and experiences of individuals to understand the complexity of the advantages and disadvantages they face within systems of power, privilege, and oppression. In individuals with multiple identities, some identities afford advantages, and others lead to being marginalized or disadvantaged (Crenshaw, 2019). In culturally heterogeneous groups, competent clinicians will be attentive to the safety and inclusivity of members of diverse identities and recognize the detrimental impact of microaggressions and exclusion, and the necessity to engage in preventative practices.

When treating members of a culturally homogeneous group, clinicians must be vigilant to avoid implicit and explicit biases that might inhibit, repress, or oppress group members. In addition to addressing the power and privilege dynamics that relate to race and ethnicity, gender, sexuality, or physical disabilities, clinicians must be sensitive to the possible presence of shame and the associated reluctance of a group member to disclose differences in opinion, beliefs, and behavior within a culturally homogenous context.

Matching clinicians and group members for culture and ethnicity generally increases the likelihood of success but is not essential. Any clinician who maintains a stance of respectful exploration can enter into a therapeutic collaboration with a homogeneous group to inspire dialogue and healing. While a clinician who identifies as a member of the same community may have the advantage of cultural familiarity, it is always best to maintain a position of attention and curiosity to avoid collusion and prejudices that can impede positive group dynamics (Rigg & Kivlighan, 2022).

Implications For Training and Practice

According to Jones et al. (2013), a culturally competent practitioner exhibits proficiency in three domains of competence: 1) beliefs and attitudes; 2) knowledge; and 3) skills. The ability to recognize personal beliefs and attitudes about others who may be perceived as different, including race, culture, ethnicity, gender identity, sexual orientation, and other variations of diversity, requires an internal process that begins with self-awareness. With good self-understanding and openness to different perspectives, practitioners can develop their knowledge and understanding of other cultural groups and develop particular skills to administer culturally sensitive psychological assessments and interventions.

In group therapy with religious members, a common feature of resistance is shame and hesitation to admit to religious noncompliance. Rubin (2011) identifies four practice principles for addressing taboo topics in group psychotherapy that would evoke feelings of shame: 1) The group facilitator must accept and carry out the responsibility to help the group raise and examine the difficult topics. 2) A group leader must be self-aware and engage in ongoing self-examination to recognize his or her own discomfort and any reactions to those discomforts.

3) A group leader can capitalize on his or her own reluctance to raise taboo topics. 4) Adopting the approach of tackling taboo topics in the group ultimately empowers practitioners.

In the reported vignette, the therapist's familiarity with the various dimensions of Orthodox Jewish culture enabled him to identify and address a group member's shame in consideration of Rubin's principles. As a member of the same homogeneous group, the therapist was sensitive to the religious concerns of group members and their inhibition of openly disclosing cultural wrongdoings. The therapist's cultural awareness enabled him to facilitate frank conversations and process the group's traumatic reaction to the experience of shame in the context of group treatment.

A therapist's ability to integrate relevant diversity factors into his or her theoretical approach to assessment and intervention is essential for the successful outcome of therapy (Fuertes et al., 2006). To treat religious clients, a culturally competent clinician will become familiar with the nuances of religious experience and be sensitive to the possible implications of observance and disobedience. To begin with, culturally skilled therapists must become aware of how their own cultural experiences, attitudes, values, and biases influence psychological processes before they become sensitive to the client's worldview and are capable of providing empathic treatment (Sue et al., 1998).

Conclusion: An Unsacred Silence

Not all silence is golden. When used as a tool in the context of individual psychotherapy, therapists can utilize silence to facilitate client reflection, challenge a client to take responsibility, facilitate a client's expression of feelings, or give themselves time to decide how to respond to their clients (Ladany et al. 2004). In group psychotherapy, the determinants of silence are more complex. Gans and Counselman (2000) address various forms, uses, and meanings of silence in group psychotherapy, and describe the absence of speech as a "powerful communication tool" that is often mistaken for inactivity. In contrast with constructive silences, Brown (2008) describes counterproductive silences in group psychotherapy that produce potentially harmful projections, transference, fears, intense negative emotions, and hostility. When facing the potential of humiliation and shame, Rutan and colleagues (2014) describe the silent group member as assuming the cautionary role to prevent the disclosure of secrets and fears that other group members may share and wish to conceal. The sounds of silence in group interactions are often louder than words.

Since silence typically conceals shame, it is vital for a culturally competent clinician to recognize the possibilities of humiliation and guilt that lurk in the cultural experiences of group participants. Rumbi (2022) examines the shame that drives the rite of confession of guilt and sin in the Toraja tradition of South Sulawesi, Indonesia and the feelings of collective shame in Toraja culture that arises when a family member or community member in a village commits a violation, primarily of moral ethics. In Judaism too, there is a concept of collective responsibility that unites individuals within the historical community of Israel (Gottlieb, 1974). During the High Holidays, a prayer called *Viddui*, which means "confession," is repeated multiple times and includes an alphabetical acrostic of various sins. The prayer is recited in first-person plural tense because the accountability and fates of community members are considered to be intertwined (My Jewish Learning, n.d.).

While prayer in the first-person plural tense helps to unite worshippers and inspire contrition in synagogue, the dread of disgrace in religiously and culturally homogeneous interpersonal process groups can contribute to a conspiracy of silence among members that compromises the therapeutic process. In the reported case example, when Baruch disclosed his "loneliness, humiliation, and regret" for failing to fulfill religious and cultural expectations, he was met initially with a combined silence that confirmed his isolation. The group's empathic failure was rooted in their shared cultural experience and collective discomfort which resulted in an enactment of their religiocultural adaptation to shame.

As an adaptive emotional response, guilt can motivate an individual to acknowledge misdeeds and rectify wrongdoings. Alternatively, when exaggerated and inhibiting, guilt can also lead to pathology and distress (Bruno et al., 2009). Baruch's desire to disclose his emotions in order to alleviate feelings of guilt coupled with his hesitation to do so out of fear of humiliation may have been rooted in an internal conflict regarding how to cope with worry. The biblical verse "Anxiety in a man's heart weighs him down, but a good word makes him glad" (English Standard Version Bible, 2001, Prov. 12:25) employs the Hebrew verb "yashchena" which can paradoxically imply both disclosure and dismissal. In their silence, the Orthodox Jewish therapist and group members may have been expressing a cultural ambivalence toward self-disclosure compounded with a learned emotional response to guilt and shame that has an unhelpful impact towards their goal of connecting to others.

Within an amalgam of ritual, mythological, doctrinal, ethical, and social expectations, the lived experience of Orthodox Judaism contains elements of camaraderie and isolation, confidence and mistrust. When working with members of faith communities, a knowledgeable clinician will recognize the possible struggles of group members and be sensitive to the subtleties of the group's dynamic expressions (Pargament & Cummings, 2010). Culturally responsive practitioners will familiarize themselves with nuances of the subculture of group participants to better hear what is spoken and what is not being said.

References

Abernethy, A. D., Grannum, G. D., & Allen, D. F. (2019). Spirituality and transformation in a community-based group in the Bahamas. *Mental Health, Religion & Culture, 22*(3), 227–243. https://doi.org/10.1080/13674676.2019.1579177.

Abernethy A. D. & Lancia, J. J. (1998). Religion and the psychotherapeutic relationship. Transferential and countertransferential dimensions. *The Journal of Psychotherapy Practice and Research, 7,* 281–289.

Agius, E. & Chircop, L. (1998). *Caring for future generations: Jewish, Christian and Islamic perspectives.* Adamantine Press Limited.

American Group Psychotherapy Association. (2023). *AGPA Guidelines for creating affirming group experiences.* AGPA.org. Retrieved June 26, 2023, from www.agpa.org/home/media/social-issue-policy-resolutions/agpa-guidelines-for-creating-affirming-group-experiences.

American Psychological Association. (2003). Guidelines on multicultural education, training, research, practice, and organizational change for psychologists. *The American Psychologist, 58*(5), 377–402. https://doi.org/10.1037/0003-066X.58.5.377.

Aronson, J. K., Saxe, L., Kadushin, C., Boxer, M., & Brookner, M. A. (2019). A new approach to understanding contemporary Jewish engagement. *Contemporary Jewry, 39,* 91–113. www.jstor.org/stable/45209190.

Arredondo, P., Toporek, R., Brown, S. P., Jones, J., Locke, D. C., Sanchez, J., & Stadler, H. (1996). Operationalization of the multicultural counseling competencies. *Journal of Multicultural Counseling and Development, 24*(1), 42–78. https://doi.org/10.1002/j.2161-1912.1996.tb00288.x.

Barlow, S. H. & Burlingame, G. M. (2006). Essential theory, processes, and procedures for successful group psychotherapy: Group cohesion as exemplar. *Journal of Contemporary Psychotherapy: On the Cutting Edge of Modern Developments in Psychotherapy, 36*(3), 107–112. https://doi.org/10.1007/BF02729053.

Berman, E. (2000). Sect, subsidy, and sacrifice: An economist's view of Ultra-Orthodox Jews. *The Quarterly Journal of Economics, 115,* 905–953. https://doi.org/10.1162/003355300554944.

Betancourt, J. R., Green, A. R., Carrillo, J. E., & Ananeh-Firempong, O. (2003). Defining cultural competence: A practical framework for addressing racial/ethnic disparities in health and health care. *Public Health Reports, 118(4),* 293–302. https://doi.org/10.1093/phr/118.4.293.

Billow, R. M. (2001). The therapist's anxiety and resistance to group therapy. *International Journal of Group Psychotherapy, 51*(2), 225–242. https://doi.org/10.1521/ijgp.51.2.225.49856.

Billow, R. M. (2006). The three R's of group: Resistance, rebellion, and refusal. *International Journal of Group Psychotherapy, 56*(3), 259–284.

Bix, A. S. (2020). 'Remember the Sabbath': A history of technological decisions and innovation in Orthodox Jewish communities. *History and Technology, 36*(2), 205–239. https://doi.org/10.1521/ijgp.2006.56.3.259.

Brown, N. W. (2008). Troubling silences in therapy groups. *Journal of Contemporary Psychotherapy, 38,* 81–85. https://doi.org/10.1007/s10879-007-9071-z.

Bruno, S., Lutwak, N., & Agin, M. A. (2009). Conceptualizations of guilt and the corresponding relationships to emotional ambivalence, self-disclosure, loneliness and alienation. *Personality and Individual Differences, 47*(5), 487–491. https://doi.org/10.1016/j.paid.2009.04.023.

Bulka, R. P. (1987). Guilt from, guilt towards. *Journal of Psychology & Judaism, 11*(2), 72–90.

Burlingame, G. M., McClendon, D. T., & Yang, C. (2019). Cohesion in group therapy. *Psychotherapy relationships that work: Evidence-based therapist contributions, 1,* 205–244. https://doi.org/10.1093/med-psych/9780190843953.003.0006.

Burlingame, G. M., Strauss, B., & Joyce, A. (2013). Change mechanisms and effectiveness of small group treatments. In M. J. Lambert (Ed.) *Bergin and Garfield's handbook of psychotherapy and behavior* change (640–689). John Wiley & Sons.

Cohen, A. B., Gorvine, B. J., & Gorvine, H. (2013). The religion, spirituality, and psychology of Jews. In K. I. Pargament, J. J. Exline, & J. W. Jones (Eds), *APA handbook of psychology, religion, and spirituality (Vol. 1): Context, theory, and research* (pp. 665–679). American Psychological Association. https://doi.org/10.1037/14045-037.

Cornish, M. A. & Wade, N. G. (2010). Spirituality and religion in group counseling: A literature review with practical guidelines. *Professional Psychology: Research and Practice, 41,* 398–404. https://doi.org/10.1037/a0020179.

Cornish, M. A., Wade, N. G., & Knight, M. A. (2013) Understanding group therapists' use of spiritual and religious interventions in group therapy. International *Journal of Group Psychotherapy, 63,* 572–591. https://doi.org/10.1521/ijgp.2013.63.4.572.

Cornish, M. A., Wade, N. G., Tucker, J. R., & Post, B. C. (2014). When religion enters the counseling group: Multiculturalism, group processes, and social justice. *The Counseling Psychologist, 42(5),* 578–600. https://doi.org/10.1177/0011000014527001.

Crenshaw, K. (2019). *On intersectionality: Essential writings.* The New Press.

Damianakis, T., Wilson, K., & Marziali, E. (2018). Family caregiver support groups: spiritual reflections' impact on stress management. *Aging & Mental Health, 22*(1), 70–76. https://doi.org/10.1080/13607863.2016.1231169.

Davis, A. Y. & Karo, J. B. E. (1996). *Kitzur Shulchan Aruch: A new translation and commentary.* Metsudah Publications.

Dearing, R. L. & Tangney, J. P. E. (2011). *Shame in the therapy hour.* American Psychological Association.

Dein, S. & Loewenthal, K. M. (2013). The mental health benefits and costs of Sabbath observance among Orthodox Jews. *Journal of Religion and Health, 52,* 1382–1390. https://doi.org/10.1007/s10943-013-9757-3.

Dollahite, D. C. & Marks, L. D. (2005). How highly religious families strive to fulfill sacred purposes. *Sourcebook of Family Theory and Research,* 533–541. https://scholarsarchive.byu.edu/facpub/4892.

Dyche, L. & Zayas, L. H. (1995). The value of curiosity and naivete for the cross-cultural psychotherapist. *Family Process, 34*(4), 389–399. https://doi.org/10.1111/j.1545-5300.1995.00389.x.

English Standard Version Bible. (2001). Ex. 31:12–17

Faiver, C. M., O'Brien, E. M., & Ingersoll, R. E. (2000). Religion, guilt, and mental health. *Journal of Counseling & Development, 78*(2), 155–161. https://doi.org/10.1002/j.1556-6676.2000.tb02573.x.

Forsyth, D. R. (2010). The nature and significance of groups. In R. K. Conyne (Ed.). *The Oxford handbook of group counseling,* 19–35. Oxford.

Frank, G., Bernardo, C. S., Tropper, S., Noguchi, F., Lipman, C., Maulhardt, B., & Weitze, L. (1997). Jewish spirituality through actions in time: Daily occupations of young Orthodox Jewish couples in Los Angeles. *The American Journal of Occupational Therapy, 51*(3), 199–206. https://doi.org/10.5014/ajot.51.3.199.

Fuertes, J. N., Stracuzzi, T. I., Bennett, J., Scheinholtz, J., Mislowack, A., Hersh, M., & Cheng, D. (2006). Therapist multicultural competency: A study of therapy dyads. *Psychotherapy: Theory, Research, Practice, Training, 43*(4), 480. https://doi.org/10.1037/0033-3204.43.4.480.

Gabbay, E., McCarthy, M. W., & Fins, J. J. (2017). The care of the ultra-Orthodox Jewish patient. *Journal of Religion and Health, 56,* 545–560.

Gans, J. S. & Counselman, E. F. (2000). Silence in group psychotherapy: A powerful communication. *International Journal of Group Psychotherapy, 50*(1), 71–86. https://doi.org/10.1007/s10943-017-0356-6.

Gans, J. S. & Weber, R. L. (2000). The detection of shame in group psychotherapy: Uncovering the hidden emotion. *International Journal of Group Psychotherapy, 50(3),* 381–396. https://doi.org/10.1080/00207284.2000.11491015.

Goffnett, J., Liechty, J. M., & Kidder, E. (2020). Interventions to reduce shame: A systematic review. *Journal of Behavioral and Cognitive Therapy, 30*(2), 141–160. https://doi.org/10.1016/j.jbct.2020.03.001.

Gottheil, R. & Ehrenfeld, S. (1906). Euphemisms. *In The Jewish Encyclopedia.* Retrieved from www.jewishencyclopedia.com/articles/5906-euphemism.

Gottlieb, D. (1974). Collective responsibility: Tradition. *A Journal of Orthodox Jewish Thought, 14*(3), 48–65.

Hagedorn, W. B. (2011). Using therapeutic letters to navigate resistance and ambivalence: Experiential implications for group counseling. *Journal of Addictions & Offender Counseling, 31*(2), 108–126. https://doi.org/10.1002/j.2161-1874.2011.tb00071.x.

Hahn, W. K. (1994). Resolving shame in group psychotherapy. International Journal of Group Psychotherapy, 44(4), 449–461. https://doi.org/10.1080/00207284.1994.11491251.

Hakak, Y. (2011). Psychology and democracy in the name of God? The invocation of modern and secular discourses on parenting in the service of conservative religious aims. *Mental Health, Religion & Culture, 14*(5), 433–458. https://doi.org/10.1080/13674671003793698.

Hess, E. (2014). The centrality of guilt: Working with Ultra-Orthodox Jewish patients in Israel. *American Journal of Psychoanalysis, 74*(3), 262–279. https://doi.org/10.1057/ajp.2014.23.

Heschel, A. J. (1951). *The Sabbath.* Farrar, Straus, and Giroux.

Hill, P. C., Pargament, K. I., Hood, R. W., Jr., McCullough, M. E., Swyers, J. P., Larson, D. B., & Zinnbauer, B. J. (2000). Conceptualizing religion and spirituality: Points of commonality, points of departure. *Journal for the Theory of Social Behaviour, 30,* 51–77. https://doi.org/10.1111/1468-5914.00119.

Horowitz, M. & Milevsky, A. (2020) Interpersonal processes in homogeneous group therapy with Orthodox Jewish Men in Israel: Case example and clinical application. *International Journal of Group Psychotherapy, 70*(4), 509 Heschel (1951). *The Sabbath.* Farrar, Straus, and Giroux 539. https://doi.org/10.1080/00207284.2020.1805619.

Humphreys, K, (2004). *Circles of recovery: Self-help organizations for addictions.* Cambridge University Press.

Jacques, J. R. (1998) Working with spiritual and religious themes in group therapy. *International Journal of Group Psychotherapy, 48*(1), 69–83. https://doi.org/10.1080/00207284.1998.11491522.

Jebreel, D. T., Doonan, R. L., & Cohen, V. (2018). Integrating spirituality within Yalom's group therapeutic factors: A theoretical framework for use with adolescents. *Group, 42*(3), 225–244. https://doi.org/10.13186/group.42.3.0225.

Jones, J. M., Sander, J. B., & Booker, K. W. (2013). Multicultural competency building: Practical solutions for training and evaluating student progress. *Training and Education in Professional Psychology, 7*(1), 12. https://doi.org/10.1037/a0030880.

Karp, D. A. (1992). Illness ambiguity and the search for meaning: A case study of a self-help group for affective disorders. *Journal of Contemporary Ethnography, 21*(2), 139–170. https://doi.org/10.1177/089124192021002001.

Ladany, N., Hill, C. E., Thompson, B. J., & O'Brien, K. M. (2004). Therapist perspectives on using silence in therapy: A qualitative study. *Counseling and Psychotherapy Research, 4*(1), 80–89. https://doi.org/10.1080/14733140412331384088.

Lazar, A., Kravetz, S., & Frederich-Kedem, P. (2002). The multidimensionality of motivation for Jewish religious behavior: Content, structure, and relationship to religious identity. *Journal for the scientific study of religion, 41*(3), 509–519. http://www.jstor.org/stable/1387460.

Lefforge, N. L., Mclaughlin, S., Goates-Jones, M., & Mejia, C. (2020) A training model for addressing microaggressions in group psychotherapy. *International Journal of Group Psychotherapy, 70(1)*, 1–28. https://doi.org/10.1080/00207284.2019.1680989.

Levine M., Perkins D.D., & Perkins, D.V. (2005). *Principles of community psychology: Perspectives and applications.* Oxford University Press.

Mahoney, A., Pargament, K. I., Tarakeshwar, N., & Swank, A. B. (2001). Religion in the home in the 1980s and 90s: A meta-analytic review and conceptual analyses of links between religion, marriage, and parenting. *Journal of Family Psychology, 15,* 559–596. https://doi.org/10.1037//0893-3200.15.4.559.

Marks, L. D. (2004). Sacred practices in highly religious families: Christian, Jewish, Mormon, and Muslim Perspectives. *Family Process,43*(2),217–231.https://doi.org/10.1111/j.1545-5300.2004.04302007.x.

Marks, L. D. & Dollahite, D. C. (2001). Religion, relationships, and responsible fathering in Latter-day Saint families of children with special needs. *Journal of Social and Personal Relationships*, 18(5), 625–650. https://doi.org/10.1177/0265407501185004.

Marks, L. D., Hatch, T. G., & Dollahite, D. C. (2018). Sacred practices and family processes in a Jewish context: Shabbat as the weekly family ritual par excellence. *Family Process, 57*(2), 448–461. https://doi.org/10.1111/famp.12286.

Mason-Schrock, D. (1996). Transsexuals' narrative construction of the" True Self. *Social Psychology Quarterly*, 176–192. https://doi.org/10.2307/2787018.

Maximo, S. I. (2019). A scoping review of ethical considerations in spiritual/religious counseling and psychotherapy. *Journal of Pastoral Care & Counseling, 73*(2), 124–133. https://doi.org/10.1177/1542305019848656.

McKenzie, J. G. (2016). *Guilt: Its meaning and significance.* Routledge.

Milevsky, A., & Eisenberg, M. (2012). Spiritually oriented treatment with Jewish clients: Meditative prayer and religious texts. *Professional Psychology: Research & Practice, 43,* 336–340. https://doi.org/10.1037/a0028035.

Miller, G. (2003). *Incorporating spirituality in counseling and psychotherapy: Theory and technique.* John Wiley & Sons, Inc.

My Jewish Learning. (n.d.). www.myjewishlearning.com/article/confession-vidui.

Narramore, S. B. (1974). Guilt: Where theology and psychology meet. *Journal of Psychology and Theology, 2*(1), 18–25. https://doi.org/10.1177/009164717400200103.

Nicholas, M. W. (1993). How to deal with moral issues in group therapy without being judgmental. *International Journal of Group Psychotherapy, 43*(2), 205–221. https://doi.org/10.1080/00207284.1994.11491217.

Ormont, L. R. (1992). *The Group Therapy Experience.* St. Martin's Press.

Pargament, K. I. (2007). *Spiritually integrated psychotherapy: Understanding and addressing the sacred.* Guilford Press.

Pargament, K. I. & Cummings, J. (2010). Anchored by faith: Religion as a resilience factor. In J. W. Reich, A. J. Zatura, & J. S. Halls (Eds), *Handbook of adult resilience*, 193–210. Guilford Press.

Pearce, M. J., Pargament, K. I., Oxhandler, H. K., Vieten, C., & Wong, S. (2019). A novel training program for mental health providers in religious and spiritual competencies. *Spirituality in Clinical Practice, 6*(2), 73–82. https://doi.org/10.1037/scp0000195.

Pew Forum on Religion and Public Life. (2019). *U.S. religious landscape survey.* http://religions.pewforum.org.

Post, B. C., Cornish, M. A., Wade, N. G., & Tucker, J. R. (2013). Religion and spirituality in group counseling: Beliefs and practices of university counseling center Counselors. *Journal for Specialists in Group Work, 38(4)*, 264–284. https://doi.org/10.1080/01933922.2013.834401.

Rassool, G. H. (2015). Cultural competence in counseling the Muslim patient: Implications for mental health. *Archives of Psychiatric Nursing, 29*(5), 321–325. https://doi.org/10.1016/j.apnu.2015.05.009.

Rennie, B. S. (1999). The view of the invisible world: Ninian Smart's analysis of the dimensions of religion and of religious experience. *Bulletin/CSSR, 28*(3), 63–69.

Richards, P. S. & Potts, R. W. (1995). Using spiritual interventions in psychotherapy: Practices, successes, failures, and ethical concerns of Mormon psychotherapists. *Professional Psychology: Research and Practice, 26,* 163–170. https://doi.org/10.1037/0735-7028.26.2.163.

Rigg, T. & Kivlighan, D. M. III. (2022). Examining between-group and within-group cultural conceal-ment in group therapy. *Professional Psychology: Research and Practice, 53*(3), 244–252. https://doi.org/10.1037/pro0000458.

Rose, E. M., Westefeld, J. S., & Ansley, T. N. (2001). Spiritual issues in counseling: Clients' beliefs and pref-erences. *Journal of Counseling Psychology, 48,* 61–71. https://doi.org/10.1037/0022-0167.48.1.61.

Rubin, S. (2011) Tackling taboo topics: Case studies in group work. *Social Work with Groups, 34,* 257–269. https://doi.org/10.1080/01609513.2011.558824.

Rumbi, F. P., Weismann, I. T., Ronda, D., Panggarra, R., & Camerling, Y. F. (2022). From social shame to spiritual shame: On the rite of confession of guilt and sin in Toraja. *HTS Teologiese Studies/Theological Studies, 78*(1), 7855.

Rutan, J. S., Stone, W. N., & Shay, J. J. (2014). *Psychodynamic group psychotherapy*. Guilford Press.

Scherman, N. (1981). *The Siddur: The prayer book: A new translation with halachic instructions and commentary anthologized from classical rabbinic sources: Nusach Ashkenaz.* Mesorah Publications.

Shafranske, E. P. (2013). Addressing religiousness and spirituality in psychotherapy: Advancing evidence-based professional practice. In R. Paloutzian & C. Park (Eds), *The handbook of the psychology of religion and spirituality* (595–616). Guilford Press.

Shapiro, R. (1999). Orthodox peer supervision and Orthodox group therapy: Two groups—one reli-gion. *Journal of Psychology and Judaism. 23,* 211–220. https://doi.org/10.1023/A:1024892411045.

Silverstein, R. (1995) Bending the conventional rules when treating the Ultra-Orthodox in the group setting, *International Journal of Group Psychotherapy, 45,* 237–249. https://doi.org/10.1080/00207284.1995.11490775.

Smart, N. (1969). *The religious experience of mankind*. Charles Scribners Sons. (Out of print.)

Smith-Gabai, H. & Ludwig, F. (2011). Observing the Jewish Sabbath: A meaningful restorative ritual for modern times. *Journal of Occupational Science, 18(4),* 347–355. https://doi.org/10.1080/14427591.2011.595891.

Stone, E. G. (2001). Culture, politics and group therapy: Identification and voyeurism. *Group Analysis, 34*(4), 501–514. https://doi.org/10.1177/05333160122078.

Sue, D. W., Carter, R. T., Casas, J. M., Fouad, N. A., Ivey, A. E., Jensen, M., & Vazquez-Nutall, E. (1998). *Multicultural counseling competencies: Individual and organizational development* (Vol. 11). Sage Publications.

Sue, S., Zane, N., Nagayama Hall, G. C., & Berger, L. K. (2009). The case for cultural competency in psychotherapeutic interventions. *Annual Review of Psychology, 60,* 525–548. https://doi.org/10.1146/annurev.psych.60.110707.163651.

Thompson, S. & Girz, L. (2020). Overcoming shame and aloneness: Emotion-focused group therapy for self-criticism. *Person-Centered and Experiential Psychotherapies, 19, 1–11.* https://doi.org/10.1080/14779757.2019.1618370.

Truax, P. (2002). Behavioral case conceptualization for adults. In M. Hersen, *Clinical behavior therapy: Adults and children* (3–36). John Wiley & Sons, Inc.

Wade, N. G., Post, B. C., Cornish, M. A., Vogel, D. L., & Runyon-Weaver, D. (2014). Religion and spirituality in group psychotherapy: Clinical application and case example. *Spirituality in Clinical Practice, 1*(2), 133. https://doi.org/10.1037/scp0000013.

Walker, D. F., Ahmed, S., Milevsky, A., Quagliana, H., & Bagasra, A. (2012a). Sacred texts. In D. F. Walker and W. L. Hathaway (Eds) *Spiritual Interventions in Child and Adolescent Psychotherapy* (pp. 155–180). Washington, DC: American Psychological Association.

Walker, D. F., Doverspike, W., Ahmed, S., Milevsky, A., & Wooley, J. (2012b). Prayer. In D. F. Walker & W. L. Hathaway (Eds) *Spiritual Interventions in Child and Adolescent Psychotherapy*. Washington, DC: American Psychological Association.

Whitley, R. (2012). Religious competence as cultural competence. *Transcultural Psychiatry, 49*(2), 245–260. https://doi.org/10.1177/1363461512439088.

Whitley, R. & Jarvis, G. E. (2015). Religious understanding as cultural competence: Issues for clini-cians. *Psychiatric Times, 32*(6), 13. https://link.gale.com/apps/doc/A417738320/AONE?u=anon~1ee17126&sid=googleScholar&xid=9ac93fe3.

Wikler, M. (1986). Pathways to treatment: How Orthodox Jews enter therapy. *Social Casework, 67*(2), 113–118. https://doi.org/10.1177/104438948606700207

Wilchek-Aviad, Y. & Malka, M. (2016). Religiosity, meaning in life and suicidal tendency among Jews. *Journal of Religion and Health, 55*(2), 480–494. http://doi.org/10.1007/s10943-014-9996-y.

Wright, F. (1994). Men, shame, and group psychotherapy. *Group, 18*(4), 212–224. https://doi.org/10.1007/BF01458098.

Yalom, I. D. (1995). *The theory and practice of group psychotherapy*. Basic Books.

Yalom, I. D. & Leszcz, M. (2020). *Theory and practice of group psychotherapy* (6th Edition). Basic Books.

Yarhouse, M. A. & Beckstead, A. L. (2011). Using group therapy to navigate and resolve sexual orientation and religious conflicts. *Counseling and Values, 56*(1–2), 96–120. https://doi.org/10.1002/j.2161-007X.2011.tb01034.x

Young, J. S., Cashwell, C., Wiggins-Frame, M., & Belaire, C. (2002). Spiritual and religious competencies: A national survey of CACREP accredited programs. *Counseling and Values, 47,* 22–33. https://doi.org/10.1002/j.2161-007X.2002.tb00221.x

6 Diversity Considerations in Psychiatry Process Groups

The Medical Doctor as Trainee

Syeda Razia Haider, Seamus Bhatt-Mackin, and Meenakshi Denduluri

Introduction

Medical training is expensive, time-intensive, and filled with opportunities and challenges. In optimal cases, teaching faculty guide trainees to balance efforts to improve clinical performance with the well-being practices necessary for a career in health care while navigating professional identity formation in complex learning environments (e.g., hospitals, clinics). This complexity is present throughout training in psychiatry and equally abundant in residency process groups (Bhatt-Mackin & Denduluri, 2023). At present, there is minimal literature on diversity dynamics in psychiatry trainee process groups, which is a major gap in the literature. This chapter is written with multiple audiences in mind: novice psychiatrist process group leaders, non-psychiatrist process group leaders, experienced process group leaders across professional disciplines, and program directors. As such, some sections may be more or less pertinent based on the reader's vantage point. Contents include sections on diversity issues in academic medicine and psychiatry, the pathway to becoming a psychiatrist in the U.S., the standard practice of psychiatry process groups, vignettes to illustrate core concepts and interventions, ethical considerations, and implications for training and practice.

Conceptual Framework

Diversity Issues in Academic Medicine and Psychiatry

Medicine is a historically white male occupation in the U.S. with structural racism woven into its fabric. From Dr. Samuel Cartwright's concept of "drapetomania" used to validate slavery in 1851 (White, 2002) to the Tuskegee Syphilis Study in the 20th century (Centers for Disease Control, 2022) to bias in psychiatric diagnosis (Snowden, 2003), organized medicine and psychiatry have repeatedly been "wrong on race" in medical school (Tweedy, 2020), residency training, and clinical practice. According to a 2019 report from the American Association of Medical College, most active physicians are White (56 percent) and male (64 percent). Black, Hispanic and Native American physicians account for about 11 percent of all practicing physicians, despite accounting for a third of the U.S. population (U.S. Census Bureau QuickFacts, n.d.) This disparity is also true in psychiatry departments, as illustrated by reports from trainees in psychiatry residencies (DeSouza et al., 2021), in essays from clinical teaching faculty (Forrester et al., 2021), and by empirical data: underrepresented minorities (URM) comprise 16 percent of psychiatry resident physicians (Wyse et al., 2020), with 2018 residency cohorts composed of approximately 52 percent White residents and 51 percent male residents (Moran, 2021).

DOI: 10.4324/9781003455783-8

Medicine struggles to retain URM trainees through a "leaky pipeline" (Barr, 2008). Studies have shown that URM undergraduate students have a disproportionate decline in interest in continuing premedical education (Barr, 2008), URM students in Undergraduate Medical Education (medical school) receive lower grades on clinical rotations (Lee et al., 2007) and URM residents are more likely to withdraw or be dismissed from Graduate Medical Education (GME) training programs (McDade, 2019). In the GME learning environment, minoritized residents experience microaggressions, report challenges negotiating personal and professional identity, and get tasked with labor as ambassadors above-and-beyond standard duties (Osseo-Asare et al., 2018). Minoritized faculty members at academic institutions have described "feelings of invisibility, lack of mentorship, lack of direct support from leadership, coping with the burden of microaggressions, and voicelessness" (Forrester, 2020). This lack of representation has a direct impact on minoritized residents through social isolation and lack of mentorship (Osseo-Asare et al., 2018). These phenomena can emerge in residency process groups. Pertinent examples are reviewed in vignettes.

Learning From Experience in Medicine and Psychiatry

Experiential learning is an organizing principle in the U.S. medical education system. This principle derives from the works of Dewey, Knowles, Kolb, and Vygotsky, among others. In *Experience and Education*, Dewey (1938) described progressive learning theory, where we learn by building on prior experiences and using them as an "organizing focus for lifelong learning and development." Knowles (1980), in describing andragogy, states that "people attach more meaning to learnings they gain from experience than those they acquire passively." Kolb (1984) asserts that learning is "a process whereby knowledge is created through the transformation of experience." He builds on Dewey's work and describes four stages of experiential learning: Concrete Experience, Reflective Observation, Abstract Conceptualization, and Active Experimentation. This type of experiential learning is progressively important for physicians as they move from medical school through residency/fellowship to unsupervised clinical practice (Yardley et al., 2012).

In medical school and residency training, the focus on "concrete experience" is shaped by the slogan "See one, Do one, Teach one" (Cameron, 1997; Kotsis & Chung, 2013). This is most often applied to common procedural skills like learning to draw blood or to place an intravenous line. This dictum prioritizes witnessing, doing, and sharing, and it appears in learning across a range of practices from lumbar puncture ('spinal tap') to giving news of a poor prognosis to de-escalating an agitated patient. Notably, "See one, Do one, Teach one" does not involve any didactics, ongoing guidance, or quality control. Although it is true that there is a move toward ongoing deliberate practice as the gold standard in medical education (Donoghue et al., 2021), this tradition is still present in explicit and implicit ways.

In most medical schools, third-year medical students rotate through different "clerkships," during which they gain skills in taking patient histories and documentation in the medical record by shadowing experienced physicians and practicing those skills with real patients. Medical students then progress to "sub-internships" in the fourth year, where they function as the first-line 'doctor-in-training' by managing the care of a small number of patients. After graduating from medical school, trainees move on to a residency training program. First-year residents are called interns, and the "first-call" providers, typically on inpatient wards. They work as part of a team, supervised by more senior residents and by attending physicians who have completed their residency training and are board-certified in a medical specialty. Attending physicians and senior residents provide teaching and mentorship to more junior residents.

General adult psychiatry residency is four years. The intern year includes six months of internal medicine/neurology and six months of acute care psychiatry rotations (inpatient, emergency, consultation–liaison). Psychiatry residents continue to gain skills in working with these sick patients during the second year of training. Residents are expected to perform patient interviews and develop plans for patient management. Attending physicians are immediately available on-site. The latter two years of psychiatry residency training usually involves working in outpatient psychiatry. Here, residents are provided with an increased level of autonomy as they gain more independence. Many psychiatry trainees come into the last two years of residency, and into psychotherapy spaces in particular, with focus on the biomedical model and a limited background in psychology. Personal psychotherapy is not a requirement or expectation, and few residents seek personal psychotherapy as a part of their training, despite the perception by many resident training directors that this practice is beneficial (Habl et al., 2010).

The Accreditation Council for Graduate Medical Education (ACGME) sets and monitors professional educational standards. These include requirements for residency training programs and behavioral markers to assess the progress of individual residents (called ACGME "Milestones") in six areas called 'core competencies' (Professionalism, Patient Care and Procedural Skills, Medical Knowledge, Practice-based Learning and Improvement, Interpersonal and Communication Skills, and Systems-based Practice; see Figure 6.1 and Figure 6.2). This includes demonstrating competency in brief and long-term supportive, psychodynamic, and cognitive-behavioral therapy (Accreditation Council for Graduate Medical Education (2022)

Patient Care 4: Psychotherapy
A: Establishes therapeutic alliance and manages boundaries
B: Selects, sets goals, and provides psychotherapies including supportive, psychodynamic, and cognitive-behavioral
C: Manages therapeutic process

Level 1	Level 2	Level 3	Level 4	Level 5
Establishes a working relationship with patients demonstrating interest and empathy	Establishes a bounded therapeutic alliance with patients with uncomplicated problems	Establishes and maintains a therapeutic alliance with patients with uncomplicated problems, and can recognize and avoid boundary violations	Establishes and maintains therapeutic alliance with patients with complicated problems, and can anticipate and appropriately manage boundary violations	Assesses and can help repair troubled alliances and/or boundary difficulties between junior residents and their patients
Lists the three core psychotherapies	Uses the common factors of psychotherapy in providing supportive therapy to patients	Provides selected psychotherapies (including supportive, psychodynamic, and cognitive-behavioral), sets goals and integrates therapy with other treatment modalities	Selects appropriate psychotherapeutic modality based on case formulation, tailors the therapy to the patient, and provides psychotherapy (at least supportive and one of psychodynamic or cognitive-behavioral) to complex patients	Tailors psychotherapeutic treatment based on awareness of own skill sets, strengths, and limitations
Accurately identifies patient emotions, particularly sadness, anger, and fear	Identifies and reflects the core feelings and key issues for the patient during the session	Identifies and reflects the core feelings, key issues and what the issues mean to the patient during the session, while managing the emotional content and feelings elicited	Identifies and reflects the core feelings, key issues, and what the issues mean to the patient within and across sessions	Links feelings, recurrent/central themes/schemas and their meaning to the patient as they shift within and across sessions

Comments:

Not Yet Completed Level 1 ☐
Not Yet Assessable ☐

©2020 Accreditation Council for Graduate Medical Education (ACGME)

Figure 6.1 ACGME Milestone—Patient Care—Psychotherapy.

Medical Knowledge 4: Psychotherapy A: Fundamentals B: Practice and indications C: Evidence base				
Level 1	Level 2	Level 3	Level 4	Level 5
Identifies psychotherapy as an effective modality of treatment	Describes the common elements across psychotherapeutic modalities	Identifies the central theoretical principles across the three core psychotherapeutic modalities: supportive, psychodynamic, cognitive-behavioral	Explains the theoretical mechanisms of therapeutic change in each of the three core modalities	Incorporates new theoretical developments into knowledge base
Describes the basic framework of a psychotherapeutic experience	Lists the basic indications and benefits of using psychotherapy	Identifies the techniques of the three core individual psychotherapies	Compares the selection criteria and potential risks, and benefits of the three core individual psychotherapies	Demonstrates sufficient evidence-based knowledge of core individual therapies to teach others
Lists the three core psychotherapy modalities	Describes the evidence for one core psychotherapy modality	Summarizes the evidence base for the three core individual psychotherapies	Analyzes the evidence base for combining psychotherapy and pharmacotherapy	
☐	☐	☐	☐	☐	☐	☐	☐	☐
Comments:				
			Not Yet Completed Level 1 ☐ Not Yet Assessable ☐	

Figure 6.2 ACGME Milestone—Medical Knowledge—Psychotherapy.

for residents to complete and graduate. There is research on teaching methods, assessment tools, and resources (Sudak et al., 2003). However, the term "competence" is not defined, and this results in wide variability across psychiatry residency programs with regard to training in psychotherapy (Sudak & Goldberg, 2012).

Psychiatry trainees are expected to learn about cultural competence as well. Projections estimate that minoritized groups will comprise over 50 percent of the U.S. population by the 2050s (Passel, 2008). To address the needs of an increasingly diverse population, the ACGME developed and implemented requirements for cultural competence in trainees (Corral et al., 2017) which are distributed across the Milestones. In psychiatry, these requirements are most often met using a combination of textbooks, supplemental reading material, traditional didactics (Corral et al., 2017), and assessment during clinical practice (ACGME Program Requirements for Graduate Medical Education in Psychiatry, 2022). In some cases, work in developing cultural competence includes experiential learning (Guzder & Rousseau, 2013; Willen, 2013; Willen & Carpenter-Song, 2013).

Learning from Experience in Group Psychotherapy

Group psychotherapy has a long tradition of learning in experiential groups. This can happen through participation in group psychotherapy or other forms of experiential group learning. When expert group psychotherapists were surveyed, they emphasized the role of experiential training in their professional development (Hahn et al., 2022).

One example is the "process group," defined as a small group which studies its own behavior to enable its members to learn about group dynamics, individual dynamics, and interpersonal communication (Swiller, 2011).

If one has not participated in a process group, it is difficult to convey the nature of the experience. Brown (2003), after reviewing the literature, proposed a synthetic definition of group process as the "here-and-now experience in the group that describes how the group is functioning, the quality of the relationships between and among members and with the leader, the emotional experiences and reactions of the group, and the group's strongest desires and fears" (p. 288). In order for members to speak to this, there must be sufficient psychological safety in a robust container and the process group leader helps this by attending to important structural components—where the group meets, at what time, and who will participate. In addition, the process group leader develops a set of agreements to which all members must assent. These group agreements influence the behavioral norms and ethical approaches that develop. However, the process group leader does not direct the content by offering prompts for discussion. Depending on the model, this can create an anxiety-inducing situation which calls for self-activation.

In this crucible, many core processes described in group dynamics can emerge and be seen in greater clarity over time. These include the stages of group development, psychological safety, group roles, and group cohesion. It is not possible for the leader of any small group to dictate—by fiat, as an authoritarian—these emergent properties which actually require the group to unfold. In addition, the stresses and support available to group members becomes more apparent to trainee group therapists through their participation in an experiential group.

This kind of learning cannot be done through reading or imagination; it is necessary to actively participate. The American Group Psychotherapy Association (AGPA) holds an annual conference with two-day process groups across a range of experience level from novice first-timers to highly experienced group therapists (Continuing ED—Meetings—Events—Training, n.d.). In addition, there are local AGPA affiliate group psychotherapy societies present through the U.S., which offer process group experiential training. Lastly, there are often training groups for group psychotherapists offered by experienced and skilled group therapists in community, university, or private practice.

Process Groups in Psychiatry Training

Many psychiatry training programs offer "process groups" for their residents. In the most recent comprehensive published report by Gans et al. (1995), less than half of the responders to surveys of psychiatry residency programs reported including T-groups (48 programs out of a total of 101). Similar results were seen in a more recent smaller survey by Khawaja et al. (2011) (seven programs out of a total of 18). Despite this, there is minimal literature on psychiatry process groups and the term "process group" is ambiguous. These groups draw from multiple conceptual traditions including psychotherapy groups, experiential process groups in allied professional fields (psychology, social work), T-groups, support groups, Balint groups, and social systems theory-based groups. Understanding the nature of psychiatry training process groups and how they differ from psychotherapy groups is essential for process group leaders.

Unlike a psychotherapy group, where the primary task is to decrease psychological suffering, a psychiatry residency process group aims to increase residents' awareness of group dynamics and interpersonal or self-in-the-group dynamics and provide support during the rigors of psychiatry training (See Table 6.1 below, adapted from Bhatt-Mackin & Denduluri, 2023). While interactions outside the group are discouraged in psychotherapy groups, they are inevitable during psychiatry residency process groups as residents have meaningful relationships with each other outside the group. The group leader in a psychotherapy group is usually a trained psychotherapist, whereas the group leader for a psychiatry training

Table 6.1 Comparison between Psychotherapy Group and Process Group Outcomes During Training in Psychiatry

	Psychotherapy Group	*Psychiatry Training Process Group*
Primary Goal(s)	Decrease psychological suffering	1. Increase awareness and knowledge of interpersonal and group dynamics 2. Provide support during the rigors of psychiatry training
Leader	Group psychotherapist	Faculty member with no supervisory, evaluative or leadership role
Group Composition	Selected by group therapist	Selected by training program
Members	Patients in treatment	Trainees in Psychiatry
Participation	Voluntary	Required or Elective
Meeting Time and Location	Determined by group therapist	Determined by training program
Interventions	Dependent on the psychotherapy type	Primarily here-and-now Discourage interpretations related to childhood or individual history Bridge cognitive & affective streams Group-as-a-whole
Outside interactions	Discouraged	Inevitable

process group is a faculty member who ideally has no supervisory, evaluative, or leadership role within the residency program so as to minimize multiple relationships. Additionally, the group leader has no role in selecting group participants in psychiatry training process groups. In fact, the program itself has influence but not the final say in who joins any particular residency class. The process group leader may have little influence in the meeting time and location, though this can depend on the relationship between the process group leader and the program director. The frame is set by program leadership. Hence, group members can include residents from one year or multiple years, voluntary or mandatory participants and run for one or multiple years.

Process groups have numerous advantages for psychiatry residents. They offer an opportunity for residents to observe senior group leaders at work (Swiller, 2011), gain the experience of being in a group, and increase awareness of their own interpersonal dynamics.

Experiential Process Group Interventions

Process group interventions draw from multiple other groups focused on clinician training. A process group that provides "good-enough" psychological support can help trainees lean on each other. Additionally, these groups can serve as a place for residents to discuss difficult patient interactions, similar to Balint groups (Mahoney et al., 2013) which Michael and Enid Balint developed in the 1950s to improve understanding of doctor-patient relationships through discussing a case example. Residency process groups can also improve residents' understanding of their own interpersonal and group relationships by maintaining a "here-and-now" focus similar to the T-group methodology that was developed by Lewin at the National Training Laboratory. While the focus of T-groups has moved into organizational consulting, Lewin believed that "learning was best accomplished when the student experienced how his or her behavior impacted others" (Highhouse, 2002) and initially developed

T-groups to address intergroup tensions, social injustice, and progressive societal change. Process group leaders can also use the group-as-a-whole to promote systems level thinking, such as Tavistock or system-centered approaches.

In summary, there are four types of groups that influence psychiatry training process groups: T-groups, support groups, group relations and Balint groups (Figure 6.3). Group interventions in psychiatry training process groups are primarily here-and-now focused. They discourage interpretations related to childhood or individual history to maintain this focus. Group-as-a-whole interactions are prioritized over those focused on individual relationships. They work towards deepening understanding of difficult clinical cases and bridging cognitive and affective streams.

Whether or not explicit attention is brought to them, diversity dynamics are present in any teaching on the subject (Forrester, 2020; Willen, 2013) and will emerge in residency process groups. Minoritized residents may be consciously or unconsciously called upon in a disproportionate way (minority tax) and may encounter microaggressions isomorphic with racism, sexism, homophobia, and other biases present in the larger society. Residents might come into the training program with different levels of comfort discussing diversity dynamics. Individuals targeted by microaggressions are harmed whether they choose to respond or not. Since participants in a residency process group are also co-workers, this can translate to conflict that impacts clinic work outside the group.

Because there is minimal literature on diversity dynamics in residency process groups (Aveline, 1993; Gans et al., 1995; Khawaja et al., 2011; Munich, 1993; Sunderji et al. 2013; Swiller, 2011) recommendations for interventions come from multiple sources. Sources include addressing diversity dynamics in psychotherapy groups (Kaklauskas & Nettles,

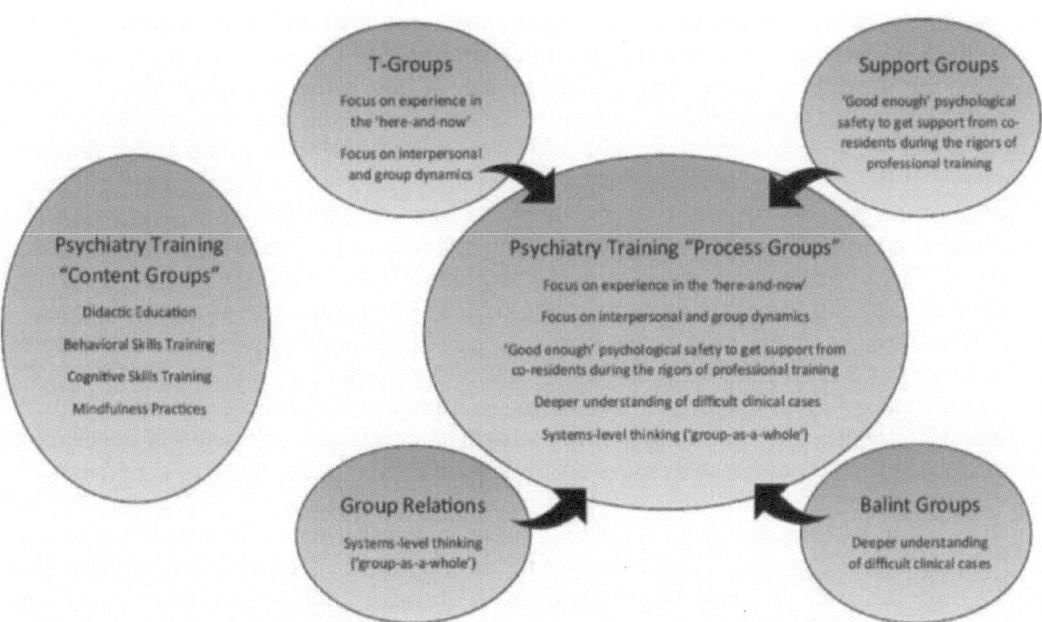

Figure 6.3 Illustration of How Psychiatry Process Groups Incorporate Features of Other Groups Focused on Clinician Training.

2020; Ribeiro, 2020), Multicultural Orientation (Kivlighan & Chapman, 2018; Kivlighan et al., 2019), training in responding to microaggressions generally (Lefforge et al., 2020) as well as in the form of cultural ruptures (Miles et al., 2021), psychotherapy supervision in psychology (Hardy, 2016; Hook et al., 2016; Jones et al., 2019) and psychiatry (DeSouza et al., 2021), process groups in non-psychiatric professional fields (Haber & Deaton, 2019; Shumaker et al., 2011), and the group relations tradition (McRae & Short, 2009).

Training Examples (Vignettes)

In this section, we use a series of brief training vignettes which we have created *de novo* to describe core background concepts and experiential process group interventions. Vignettes are organized by a focused area of process group leadership: working in the larger system, building a working relationship with the training director, co-leadership in the process group, broaching social identity, scapegoating, microaggressions and each vignette offers interventions for a process group leader to consider.

Vignette #1

A community-based White cis-male identifying heterosexual psychiatrist and group psychotherapist is contacted by a training program administrator in the psychiatry residency of a prestigious academic medical center and invited to take on the resident process group. Recalling a positive experience of process groups during his own professional development, this community clinician is pleased and eager to get involved. After communicating interest, he does not hear more information for three months, when he receives notice that the process group will happen in a few weeks. Concerned about the dearth of communication, the group therapist reaches out and requests a meeting to get more information and begin to develop a working relationship. The meeting happens, but it is again with a busy program administrator, who does not have any experience with process groups. During this meeting, the community clinician learns that the residency program had a process group in the remote past, that there is a new White cis-female identifying chair of the department who suggested a process group to the experienced Black cis-female identifying program director; and the program director has not herself had any experience with a process group. The community clinician receives two emails later in the day: 1) the program director expresses hope that the process group will help foster cross-racial dialogue, as two URM psychiatry residents transferred away from the program in the most recent two years and 2) the department chair thanks the community clinician for taking on the process group, reflecting on their own positive process group experience with a senior and nationally famous group therapist. The community clinician is now quite anxious and uncertain how to proceed. The ambivalence of this system is palpable.

Discussion: Process groups often cannot happen unless there is interest and support from the training program director. In addition, it is vital to discuss and decide on the learning goals for the process group. While it is uncommon for a process group to create a new problem that is not already present in the larger system, it is also highly unlikely that a process group will solve such problems. In this situation, there is a wish for change regarding URM resident retention. However, if the process group is the only strategy used to address underlying issues, the endeavor is destined to disappoint, as it will necessarily not include the residents who left, so there isn't any serious attempt to assess their concerns. In addition, the framing of the process group as an intervention to solve a systemic problem focuses on the individual residents and their experience of discontent and suffering (an individualistic target of change), instead of addressing aspects of the system that perpetuated any harm to the two residents who left the program.

Medical training can happen in suboptimal learning environments, despite the difficulties involved, and psychiatry process groups can happen suboptimally, too. However, given the complexity of these dynamics, it would be wise for this community clinician process group leader to request the department support co-leaders in the process group. Co-leadership allows for greater representation of social identities in the leadership team, including the intersection of dominant and nondominant identities. In addition, in the case of this vignette, there are definite advantages of working with a co-leader who is already part of this system. This could give the "binocular view" favored by organizational consultants—the community therapist can view process group dynamics as an outsider with limited access to the unstated context, while the co-leader can view the same dynamics with context in the forefront of their mind. For example, with regard to resident departures, the community therapist will have an outsider view, while his co-leaders might have some insider-based hypotheses. As with any process group leader, it is vital that the co-leader inside the system is not a direct supervisor or in any other evaluative position in relation to the psychiatry residents in the process group; this is an important ethical boundary to hold.

Vignette #2

A group of ten psychiatry interns meet for their first process group session. The group consists of six cis-women, five Black, Indigenous, People of Color (BIPOC), and three residents who identify as LGBTQIA+. The interns have known each other for two weeks and interacted in other professional settings outside the process group. The group leaders who had no other relationship to the residency program include a cis-male, heterosexual, white psychologist in his 70s and a cis-woman, white, bisexual psychologist in her late 30s. When the group leaders introduce themselves, they focus on their professional identities and experience running psychiatry process groups, each giving their full title, first name and last name, with no self-disclosure of racial identity, pronouns or any other aspect of their social identity. In addition, they do not reveal that the younger psychologist has substantially more experience leading process groups and this is the first time that the older psychologist has lead a process group.

The co-leaders are new to each other, so they meet ahead of starting their work in the process group and agree to alternate starting the meeting, each doing so in their own way. The younger cis-female wonders aloud to signal the group's beginning by stating "I'm curious about how we will begin our work today" and the older cis-male psychologist started by noting the number of meetings that have been completed (e.g., "This is the fourth meeting of this process group") or the number of meetings that remain (e.g., "There are five meetings left in this process group, including today.")

At the eighth meeting, a white cis-male intern notices the difference in approach that each leader takes. As he did so, he refers to the cis-female psychologist by her first name ("Jane") and he refers to the cis-male psychologist by his title and last name ("Dr. Roberts"). The group does not work with this intern's observation and does not speak to the difference in appellation. Neither co-leader intervenes. Over the next three meetings, it becomes a behavioral norm for group members to refer to the co-leaders in these discrepant ways. At this point, the co-leaders observe the different way that the group is relating to them. After some examination of the here-and-now, their observation is followed by a flood of emotional sharing of experiences from cis-female interns about the sexist interactions with patients, supervisors, and fellow trainees. Several weeks later, this process group was also able to expand beyond a simple gender binary to allow for a broader range of gender experiences, such as non-binary.

Discussion: Visible and acknowledged differences between the co-leaders allowed for the emergence in the process group of a process that is also ongoing in the training environment; gender bias is present in this process group and it continues to be present in the health care setting. In this case, the new co-leader team was caught a bit off-guard and delayed responding until they had more information about what was happening in this group. In this case, because other group members joined, there was a subgroup or whole group dynamic at work. It may have worked to their advantage to address the issue when there were multiple members carrying it. However, if the group leaders completely avoided addressing it, then the group would be unlikely to be able to contain this basic difference.

To intervene, the co-leaders could speak to the group-as-a-whole (e.g., "I wonder what it is about this process group in this particular context that one co-leader is addressed as "Doctor Robert" and the other is addressed as "Jane"). The group leaders could speak to a specific member and reference a whole group process, such that the comment is heard by all present (e.g., "I noticed that you—and some of your colleagues—are using different levels of formality with each of us—I wonder what that means?"). Finally, the co-leaders could have a conversation between themselves in the presence of the group without specifically addressing their comments to anyone in particular (e.g., "Have you noticed how the group members call me "Doctor Robert" and they call you "Jane"?). There are pros and cons of each approach and factors to consider include the level group cohesion, the developmental stage, and the robustness of the co-leader team.

Vignette #3

Consider the same process group as the second example. However, when the leaders introduce themselves, they explicitly acknowledge their privileged (white, cis-gender, and able-bodied) and marginalized identities. One group leader introduces the first process group session in this manner: "Hello everyone, welcome to process group. As we discussed in the orientation sessions, we will be examining group dynamics in the moment as they arise. But first let's go around and introduce ourselves. As part of our work together, Robert and I will invite people to consider how aspects of our identities also impact how we participate in the process group and come into this space. My name is Jane Goodman—I am a psychologist, I identify as white, a cis-woman, and able-bodied." The co-leader adds, "Yes, Jane and I are very excited to be your process group leaders. My name is Robert, I am also a psychologist by training, and I identify as white, a cis-man, and able-bodied. There are some aspects of our identity that diverge—which allows for us to see from different vantage points—and others which do not. In the areas in which we are most similar, we are at the greatest risk for limitations in what we will notice. We'll do our best to stay open to what we could be missing."

Discussion: There is value in group leaders explicitly disclosing different aspects of their identities. By "broaching" the conversation and "going first" group leaders can create a space for group members to reflect on their own privileged and marginalized identities. This can help in creating a group norm around discussing diversity dynamics which will have a downstream impact on the group's development.

Vignette #4

A process group contains the entirety of a nine resident PGY3 cohort, and it happens in parallel with a didactic seminar on group psychotherapy in which eight members participate. In the seminar, a White cis-male identifying teaching attending psychiatrist provides readings on the psychodynamic approach to understanding scapegoating in therapy groups, focusing on how the scapegoated member "volunteers" for the role, on an unconscious level, based on prior experiences in childhood and family life. Multiple members of the residency cohort are international medical graduates (IMG); however, only one member who is an IMG objects to the singular focus on personality as a primary factor in scapegoating process, stating their belief that visible, identity-related differences can also contribute to this process. The teaching attending dismisses this as a possibility.

The following day, the group leader intervenes with conscious intention to illuminate a whole-group process in the group ("Pairing dynamics can only succeed in containing anxiety in the short-term") but which singles out one resident who happens to be separating from their romantic partner (a person not in the process group). The typically vocal resident—who had objected in the scapegoating didactic—now challenges the whole-group intervention, believing themselves to be coming to the defense of the absent member ("Many people long for deep partnerships that require pairing!"). Other group members consciously "know" about their co-resident's separation but somehow forget in the moment and express irritation with the challenge ("You're always questioning everything!"), devalue the objection ("That doesn't have anything to do with what we are doing!") and then ignore subsequent contributions from this member, despite multiple silent group members agreeing with the objection. The process group leader does not intervene further as this scapegoating process unfolds.

Discussion: Process group leaders must intentionally and actively acknowledge that foundational systems of treatment, research, and clinical education in group psychotherapy are rooted in unacknowledged racist, White supremacist and patriarchal values. Core concepts must be broadened. In addition, the 'tasks of the privileged' (Hardy, 2016) apply across the leader-member relationship. True humility is needed. Process group leaders—and group dynamics didactic teachers—need to adapt their theories and approaches to the primary educational focus of process groups. Just as the "construction of the difficult patient" can happen in therapy groups (Gans & Alonso, 1998); the construction of a difficult "learner type" can happen in educational endeavors (Forrester et al., 2021).

In this vignette, the first place of intervention is in the didactic course where a more culturally humble mindset could have helped the teaching attending to seriously consider the manner with which scapegoating is itself a culturally embedded concept with a specific historical referent. The vocal resident is providing an opportunity for expanding the knowledge base and there is a valuable research project in their objection. It might be the case that the teaching attending doesn't even quite understand the objection. And that might be the first opportunity to intervene—getting more clarification, in the didactic teaching session.

There is a second point of potential confusion in this vignette—the group-as-a-whole intervention. It takes practice to understand the purpose of the approach to process illumination. For some members, it is reassuring to include all in the responsibility for the work of the group. It is inevitable, however, that a group-as-a-whole intervention can also be taken quite personally by a member. There are a few strategies to help with this. It can be useful to provide an orientation session in which this approach is outlined didactically. It can also be useful to provide 'micro-didactics' after each meeting of the process group. These moves toward more cognitive, psycho-education approaches, especially in the process group which can be mandated, are consistent with recommendations (Brown, 2017).

Vignette #5

In a residency process group of 12 members including three international medical graduates, Farida, a Pakistani Muslim cis-woman resident, shared an upsetting incident in which a patient in the parking lot of her clinic looked at her angrily and called her an "Osama lover." In response, Josh, a white American Christian cis-man resident who has a good working rapport with the first resident laughed and said, "I've been called an Obama lover by a patient before, which is almost as bad in this part of the country." The group leader, an Indian American atheist cis-woman, raised her eyebrows and frowned in response, without verbalizing her reaction. The first resident appeared upset but did not speak for the remainder of the group.

Discussion: In this instance, a microaggression has occurred in the process group when the second resident makes light of the first resident's relaying of the patient's microaggression. He may have made this comment with the good intention of bringing humor into his co-resident's stressful situation or trying to relate; however, this was received as dismissive and invalidating by the first resident. Ideally, the group leader would be able to foster an environment where discussing cultural dynamics would be expected, recognize and name microaggressions in the moment, and provide support for the people who were microaggressed against.

For example, the group leader could have started by saying, "Let's pause for a moment—a microaggression has just occurred. Josh, it seemed like you were trying to bring in some humor, but equating Farida's experience with your experience in this instance minimizes the racism she experienced." Josh appears aghast and says, "I'm sorry, Farida, I was just trying to make you feel better, but it probably wasn't right of me to joke like that." Farida says, "Yes, I was taken aback—what I was describing was actually a really scary moment—I was shook," and went on to describe more about the incident, receiving support from her fellow process group members. In residency process groups where group members have ongoing working and personal relationships, the urge to avoid discussion of uncomfortable cultural dynamics may be stronger than in therapy groups, which underscores the importance of group leaders developing comfort with navigating such issues.

Ethical Considerations

Ethical considerations in psychiatry training process groups primarily emerge, owing to the multiple relationships between group members, program leadership and process group leaders. Residency programs are typically situated in academic medical institutions; hence, the culture of a residency program is impacted by the culture of medicine and the training program. Psychiatry training process groups can provide a platform for playing out these dynamics as discussed in some of the vignettes above. This section will discuss the ethical principles of beneficence, nonmaleficence, autonomy, and justice as it relates to diversity dynamics in psychiatry training process groups.

As previously discussed, academic medicine has a "leaky pipeline" problem. A survey of minoritized residents published in 2018 (Osseo-Asare et al.) reported that minoritized residents experienced "A Daily Barrage of Microaggressions and Bias" including the following: being treated as an "alien in one's own land", "assumption of lower status" (such as being mistaken for transport staff or nurses), "exoticization and assumptions of similarity" (such as black residents being called each other's names despite looking very different), and explicit bias. They also faced barriers to reporting these issues because of historical experiences with concerns related to diversity dynamics being unacknowledged or pushed aside. Additionally, residents may experience a fear of repercussions after reporting concerns as there were situations where the program leadership made discriminatory comments. The hectic 70–80 hour work schedules also make it difficult for residents to find time to report these concerns. Residents are not always trained to discuss dynamics related to social identity with respect to themselves (gender, race, power, etc.). It can be taxing to repeatedly give voice to a minoritized experience while trying to assimilate into a culture of medicine that remains predominantly white, male, and cis-heterosexual.

Since these dynamics deeply influence trainee experience in residency, it is inevitable that they will show up in a residency process group and it falls within the ethical principle of non-maleficence to pay attention to these issues as they directly impact the well-being of residents in the process groups. In a process group, residents may take on roles that are similar to the type of roles they assume in other settings and may be influenced by stereotypes related to different marginalized identities. These roles "emerge in groups as both defensive and adaptive mechanisms" (McRae, 2009). Minoritized group members may also experience "coercion, intimidation, microaggression and discrimination" (Barbender, 2022) in experiential groups. There may be expectations about "acceptable" ways to give voice to these issues such as holding a stance of only addressing dynamics or microaggressions when brought up by the group members. The process group leader needs to be prepared to address group dynamics that will arise in response to these systemic issues.

Residency process groups are unique in that there are over-lapping relationships that exist between residents; they are colleagues as well as group participants. Friendships and conflict outside the group can impact participation in the group. Residents might compete for chief resident positions, awards, and training opportunities outside the process group (Swiller, 2011). Additionally, peer feedback can be a part of a resident's performance evaluation in many training programs. Process groups that take place within a cohort may "stretch the interpersonal boundaries for some of the students" (Haber, 2019). "Preexisting cohort dynamics, increased exposure, and the inability to escape the group members after termination of the group" (Haber, 2019) can create barriers to discussing diversity related dynamics and make it difficult to maintain a here-and-now focus.

To maintain psychological safety in this situation, process group leaders need to be particularly mindful about confidentiality. During group orientation, the process group leader should explicitly discuss the limitations around confidentiality (such as disclosure of suicidal or homicidal ideation). To minimize the ethical concerns that may arise with the management of multiple roles (overlapping supervisory and group facilitator relationships), it is ideal if the process group leader is not otherwise involved in the residency training program. Programs should consider recruiting experienced and skilled process group leaders and compensating them for their time (Bhatt-Mackin & Denduluri, 2023). However, if this is not possible and the group leader has other evaluative roles within the training program, leaders need to ensure that the material discussed in the group will not be used for grading or disciplinary action (Haber, 2019).

Most psychiatry residents enter training with very little to no experience with process groups. To foster nonmaleficence and autonomy, an informed consent discussion that includes "a rationale, learning objectives, and group agreements for participation" prior to the start of the group is recommended (Bhatt-Mackin & Denduluri, 2023; Haber, 2019). Participation in a process group can be a source of great support for residents, but it is also laborious work. Residents have to evaluate the risks and benefits of self-disclosure when it comes to uncomfortable topics such as racial or gender dynamics. Process group participation should be voluntary, with freedom to decline participation without additional scrutiny. The group should meet at a time that is protected for this purpose so that residents do not feel obligated to attend to other work commitments.

During the COVID-19 pandemic, most residency programs shifted to virtual didactics. Many therapy groups and residency process groups shifted to the online environment as well. In these online process groups, issues of equitable access might arise. Medical school graduates have a median debt of $200,000 (Association of American Medical Colleges, n.d.) with students from low-income backgrounds being disproportionately burdened by student loan debt. This can impact access to resources necessary for participating in online groups such as a private space and reliable internet access. Residency training programs who have switched over to online process groups should ensure that residents from disadvantaged backgrounds have appropriate tools to participate in these groups.

There can be some advantages of online process groups as well, which may mitigate some of the ethical concerns related to the multiple relationships described above. Bhatt-Mackin et al. (2022) describe a novel, online, cross-residency process group that recruited residents from different residency programs. This group was structured such that there were two initial orientation/didactic sessions, eight sessions of experiential group, followed by two sessions of reflection and conclusion. This group format allowed for voluntary participation with informed consent from the participants. Additionally, since the ten participants included trainees from six different residency programs, the chances of relationships outside the group affecting in-group dynamics were minimized.

Intersectionality

It is important for process group leaders to be mindful of how social systems of power interact with each other. Most people hold multiple intersecting identities with varying levels of social privilege, which can add an extra layer of complexity to the challenges described above. For instance, trainees who belong to the same racial/ethnic groups may differ in other aspects of their identity. Trainees may hold privilege in some identities and not in others. This intersection will affect their perception of marginalization.

Consider a white physician who is a first generation college graduate and comes from a low-income background versus a BIPOC physician from a financially privileged background with two physician parents. While the second physician might have access to more resources within the field of medicine, their identity as a Person of Color means that they will face oppression from prevailing power structures. In a psychiatry training process group, this might appear as the white physician feeling disadvantaged by their socioeconomic background and being unwilling to understand the BIPOC physicians' challenges navigating the medical world. While leading process groups for trainees, it is important for group leaders to hold these varying identities without judgement, and encourage exploration of intersectionality.

Implications for Training and/or Practice

Implications for Trainees

Professional training experiences are often the foundation for subsequent clinical practice (Yardley et al., 2012). Given this fact, it is crucial to do our best from the beginning. If process groups are to remain an integral part of psychiatry training, an explicit focus on diversity dynamics is important.

"Here-and-now" interactions are inherently influenced by our past experiences and projections (Willen, 2013; Yalom & Leszcz, 2020). A residency process group with an explicit focus on diversity dynamics can provide a platform for trainees to recognize microaggressions as they happen and learn how to respond to them. Seeing cultural humility—an open and curious stance towards diversity (Kivlighan et al., 2019)—modeled by process group leaders can be a salient experience in experiential learning. The opposite can be quite detrimental for learning. Willen (2013) describes a course for psychiatry residents on "cultural sensitivity" in a New England training where "classroom-based engagement with the clinical implications of culture and difference can run awry when the emotional potency of these issues is not adequately taken into account." An experiential process group with a skilled leader can provide a platform to engage with the emotional potency of these issues.

An explicit focus on diversity dynamics in residency process groups can impact all trainees. For instance, discussions of racial dynamics can evoke strong feelings ranging from guilt to defensiveness in white participants. Discussions of these feelings in a process group during residency can lead to a deeper appreciation of such dynamics in the "real world." This can translate to improved clinician skills for working with minoritized populations.

Implications for Practice

Residency program leadership should prioritize DEIJ and recruit residents with diverse backgrounds and life experiences. Academic medicine programs should also invest efforts towards recruiting diverse faculty members to provide mentorship for young trainees. It is important for all leaders to have ongoing diversity related training, education, and consultation. This will help them aid trainees with diverse backgrounds as they experience navigating diversity dynamics in academic medicine.

As the U.S. becomes a country where People of Color comprise a majority of the population, psychiatry trainees must be prepared to adequately work with diverse patients. Integrating discussions of diversity dynamics within process groups can address an ACGME requirement for cultural competence.

Implications for the Profession

While it is true that psychiatry in the U.S. has a long road to travel with regard to inclusion, representation, and justice, efforts are underway in the area of leadership (Jordan et al., 2021; Stewart, 2021), hiring (Doyle, 2022; Liu et al, 2022), psychiatry resident recruitment (Ojo & Hairston, 2021), residency program leadership (Rohrbaugh & DeJong, 2022), and psychiatry resident empowerment (Londono Tobon et al., 2019). As a powerful experiential learning modality, process groups during psychiatry residency can stay "neutral," impede, or facilitate our collective travel. We strongly advocate for the latter and hope to add to resources available to residency program leadership, process group leaders, and psychiatry resident members with this book chapter.

Conclusion

Process groups can be an integral part of the psychiatry training experience. They incorporate methodology from different types of groups, including T-groups and support groups. Academic medicine is working towards becoming increasingly diverse and trying to fix its leaky pipeline problem. Some members and leaders in organized psychiatry are working to address structural racism to achieve diversity and inclusion in the psychiatric workforce (Sudak & Stewart, 2021). Process groups during training in psychiatry offer the opportunities and challenges which call for actively attending to diversity considerations. We have described different strategies for residency program leadership and process group leaders to facilitate exploration of these dynamics.

References

ACGME Program Requirements for Graduate Medical Education in Psychiatry. (2022). www.acgme. org/globalassets/pfassets/programrequirements/400_psychiatry_2022_tcc.pdf.

Association of American Medical Colleges. (2019). *Diversity in medicine: Facts and figures 2019*. Retrieved June 14, 2023, from www.aamc.org/data-reports/workforce/report/diversity-medicine-facts-and-figures-2019.

Association of American Medical Colleges. (n.d). *Student debt: Ensuring medical school remains affordable*. Retrieved June 15, 2023, from https://students-residents.aamc.org/advocacy/student-debt-ensuring-medical-school-remains-affordable.

Aveline, M. O. (1993). Principles of leadership in brief training groups for mental health care professionals. *International Journal Group Psychotherapy, 43*(1), 107–109. https://doi.org/10.1080/0020 7284.1994.11491208.

Barbender, V. & Macnair-Semands, R. (2022). Supervision. In *The ethics of group psychotherapy: Principles and practical strategies*. Routledge. https://doi.org/10.4324/9781003105527.

Barr, D. A., Gonzalez, M. E., & Wanat, S. F. (2008). The leaky pipeline: Factors associated with early decline in interest in premedical studies among underrepresented minority undergraduate students. *Academic Medicine: Journal of the Association of American Medical Colleges, 83*(5), 503–511. https://doi.org/10.1097/ACM.0b013e31816bda16.

Bhatt-Mackin, S. & Denduluri, M. (2023). Recommendations for implementing, leading, and participating in process groups during training in psychiatry. *Academic Psychiatry. 47,* 309–313. https://doi.org/10.1007/s40596-023-01794-6.

Bhatt-Mackin, S., Farid, N., Martinez, A., Owen, A., Mantilla-Rivas, J., & Denduluri, M. (2022). Feasibility of a novel online cross-residency group dynamics course with didactics, experiential T-group, and review [published online ahead of print, 2022 Sep 15. *Academic Psychiatry, 1–2*. https://doi.org/10.1007/s40596-022-01703-3.

Bhatt-Mackin, S. & Feiger, A. (2023). Blue ink spots: Working toward accurate self-knowledge through self-awareness. In S. G. De Golia & R. Wang (Eds), *The psychiatry resident handbook: How to thrive in training* (pp. 295–304). American Psychiatric Association Publishing.

Brown, N. (2003). Conceptualizing process. *International Journal of Group Psychotherapy. 53*(2), 225–244. https://doi.org/10.1521/ijgp.53.2.225.42814.

Brown, N. (2017). The deviant group member. *Group 41*(2), 135–146. https://doi.org/10.13186/group.41.2.0135.

Cameron, J. L. (1997). William Stewart Halsted. Our surgical heritage. *Annals of Surgery, 225*(5), 445–458. https://doi.org/10.1097/00000658-199705000-00002.

Centers for Disease Control and Prevention. (2022). *The syphilis study at Tuskegee timeline*. (2022, December 20). www.cdc.gov/tuskegee/timeline.htm.

Continuing ED—Meetings- Events—Training. (n.d.). Agpa.org. Retrieved June 15, 2023, from https://agpa.org/home/continuing-ed-meetings-events-training.

Corral, I., Johnson, T. L., Shelton, P. G., & Glass, O. (2017). Psychiatry resident training in cultural competence: An educator's toolkit. *The Psychiatric Quarterly, 88*(2), 295–306. https://doi.org/10.1007/s11126-016-9472-9.

De Golia, S. & Wang, R. (2023). *The psychiatry resident handbook: How to thrive in training*. American Psychiatric Association Publishing.

DeSouza, F., Mathis, M., Lastra, N., & Isom, J. (2021). Navigating race in the psychotherapeutic encounter: A call for supervision. *Academic Psychiatry: The Journal of the American Association of Directors of Psychiatric Residency Training and the Association for Academic Psychiatry, 45*(1), 132–133. https://doi.org/10.1007/s40596-020-01328-4.

Dewey, J. (1938). *Experience and education*. Free Press.

Donoghue, A., Navarro, K., Diederich, E., Auerbach, M., & Cheng, A. (2021). Deliberate practice and mastery learning in resuscitation education: A scoping review. *Resuscitation Plus, 6*, 100137. https://doi.org/10.1016/j.resplu.2021.100137.

Doyle, M. (2022). Disability inclusion in psychiatry: Strategies to improve and increase diversity within the psychiatrist workforce. *Psychiatric Clinics of North America, 45*(2), 279–282. https://doi.org/10.1016/j.psc.2022.03.006.

Edmondson, A. C. & Lei, Z. (2014). Psychological safety: The history, renaissance, and future of an interpersonal construct. *Annual Review of Organizational Psychology and Organizational Behavior, 1*, 23–43. https://doi.org/10.1146/annurev-orgpsych-031413-091305.

Forrester, A. (2020). Why I stay—The other side of underrepresentation in academia. *The New England Journal of Medicine, 383*(4), e24. https://doi.org/10.1056/NEJMpv2022100.

Forrester, A., Nagy, G. A., & Bhatt-Mackin, S. (2021). Learner types: Social roles encountered in multicultural clinical education in psychiatry. *Academic Psychiatry, 45*(1), 130–131. https://doi.org/10.1007/s40596-020-01387-7.

Frawley, W. (1989). Thought and language. Lev Vygotsky (A. Kozulin, revised edition). Cambridge, MA: MIT Press, 1986. pp. lxi, 287. *Studies in Second Language Acquisition, 11*(3), 331–332. https://doi.org/10.1017/S0272263100008172.

Gans, J. S. & Alonso, A. (1998). Difficult patients: Their construction in group therapy. *International Journal of Group Psychotherapy, 48*, 311–326. https://doi.org/10.1080/00207284.1998.11491545.

Gans, J. S., Rutan, J. S., & Wilcox, N. (1995). T-groups (training groups) in psychiatric residency programs: Facts and possible implications. *International Journal Group Psychotherapy, 45*(2), 169–183. https://doi.org/10.1080/00207284.1995.11490771.

Guzder, J. & Rousseau, C. (2013). A diversity of voices: The McGill "working with culture" seminars. *Culture, Medicine and Psychiatry, 37*(2), 347–364. https://doi.org/10.1007/s11013-013-9316-0.

Haber, R. & Deaton, J. (2019). Facilitating an experiential group in an educational environment: Managing dual relationships. *International Journal of Group Psychotherapy, 69*(4), 434–458. https://doi.org/10.1080/00207284.2019.1656078.

Habl, S., Mintz, D. L., & Bailey, A. (2010). The role of personal therapy in psychiatric residency training: A survey of psychiatry training directors. *Academic Psychiatry: The Journal of the American Association of Directors of Psychiatric Residency Training and the Association for Academic Psychiatry, 34*(1), 21–26. https://doi.org/10.1176/appi.ap.34.1.21.

Hahn, A., Paquin, J. D., Glean, E., McQuillan, K., & Hamilton, D. (2022). Developing into a group therapist: An empirical investigation of expert group therapists' training experiences. *The American Psychologist, 77*(5), 691–709. https://doi.org/10.1037/amp0000956.

Hardy, K. V. (2016). Mastering context talk: Practical skills for effective engagement. In T. Bobes (Ed.), *Culturally sensitive supervision and training: Diverse perspectives and practical applications.* Routledge.

Highhouse, S. (2002). A history of the T-group and its early applications in management development. *Group Dynamics: Theory, Research, and Practice, 6*(4), 277–290. https://doi.org/10.1037/1089-2699.6.4.277.

Hook, J. N., Edward Watkins, C, Jr, Davis, D. E., Owen, J., Tongeren, D. R., & Ramos, M. J. (2016). Cultural humility in psychotherapy supervision. *American Journal of Psychotherapy, 70*(2), 149–166. https://doi.org/10.1176/appi.psychotherapy.2016.70.2.149.

Johnson, A. H., Nease, D. E., Milberg, L. C., & Addison, R. B. (2004). Essential characteristics of effective Balint group leadership. *Family Medicine, 36*(4), 253–259.

Jones, C. T., Welfare, L. E., Melchior, S., & Cash, R. M. (2019). Broaching as a strategy for intercultural understanding in clinical supervision. *The Clinical Supervisor, 38*(1), 1–16. https://doi.org/10.1080/07325223.2018.1560384.

Jordan, A., Shim, R. S., & Rodriguez, C. I. (2021). Psychiatry diversity leadership in academic medicine: Guidelines for success. *American Journal Psychiatry, 178*(3), 224–228. https://doi.org/10.1176/appi.ajp.2020.20091371.

Kaklauskas, J. F. & Nettles, R. (2020). Towards multicultural and diversity proficiency as a group psychotherapist. In F. J. Kaklauskas & L. R. Greene (Eds), *Core principles of group psychotherapy: An integrated theory, research and practice training manual.* Routledge.

Khawaja, I. S., Pollock, K., & Westermeyer, J. J. (2011). The diminishing role of psychiatry in group psychotherapy: A commentary and recommendations for change. *Innovations Clinical Neuroscience, 8*(11), 20–23.

Kivlighan, D. M. & Chapman, N. A. (2018). Extending the multicultural orientation (MCO) framework to group psychotherapy: A clinical illustration. *Psychotherapy, 55*(1), 39–44. https://doi.org/10.1037/pst0000142.

Kivlighan, D. M., Drinane, J. M., Tao, K. W., Owen, J., & Liu, W. M. (2019). The detrimental effect of fragile groups: Examining the role of cultural comfort for group therapy members of color. *Journal Counseling Psychology, 66*(6), 763–770. https://doi.org/10.1037/cou0000352.

Knowles, M. S. (1980). *The modern practice of adult education: From pedagogy to andragogy*. Association Press.

Kolb, D. (1984). Experiential learning: Experience as the source of learning and development. In *Journal of Business Ethics*, *1*(2).

Kotsis, S. V. & Chung, K. C. (2013). Application of see one, do one, teach one concept in surgical training. *Plastic and Reconstructive Surgery*, *131*(5), 1194–1201. https://doi.org/10.1097/PRS.0b013e318287a0b3.

Lee, K. B., Vaishnavi, S. N., Lau, S. K. M., Andriole, D. A., & Jeffe, D. B. (2007). "Making the grade:" Noncognitive predictors of medical students' clinical clerkship grades. *Journal of the National Medical Association*, *99*(10), 1138–1150.

Lefforge, N. L., Mclaughlin, S., Goates-Jones, M., & Mejia, C. (2020). A training model for addressing microaggressions in group psychotherapy. *International Journal of Group Psychotherapy*, *70*(1), 1–28. https://doi.org/10.1080/00207284.2019.1680989.

Lewin, M. (1992). The impact of Kurt Lewin's life on the place of social issues in his work. *Journal of Social Issues*, *48*, 15–29. https://doi.org/10.1111/j.1540-4560.1992.tb00880.x.

Liu, H. Y., Larson, A. R., & Strong, S. A. (2022). Workforce diversity, equity, and inclusion: A crucial component of professionalism in psychiatry. *Psychiatric Clinics of North America*, *45*(2), 243–258. https://doi.org/10.1016/j.psc.2022.02.001.

Londono Tobon, A., Budde, K. S., & Rohrbaugh, R. M. (2019). A novel approach to fostering diversity in graduate medical education: Chief residents for diversity and inclusion. *Academic Psychiatry: The Journal of the American Association of Directors of Psychiatric Residency Training and the Association for Academic Psychiatry*, *43*(3), 344–345. https://doi.org/10.1007/s40596-019-01055-5.

Mahoney, D., Diaz, V., Thiedke, C., Mallin, K., Brock, C., Freedy, J., & Johnson, A. (2013). Balint groups: The nuts and bolts of making better doctors. *International Journal of Psychiatry in Medicine*, *45*(4), 401–411. https://doi.org/10.2190/PM.45.4.j.

McDade, W. (2019). *Diversity and Inclusion in Graduate Medical Education Chief Diversity and Inclusion Office Accreditation Council for Gradutae Medical Education*. https://southernhospitalmedicine.org/wp-content/uploads/2019/10/McDade-ACGME-SHM-Presentation-McDade-Final.pdf

McRae, M. D. & Short, E. L. (2009). *Racial and cultural dynamics in group and organizational life*. SAGE Publications.

Miles, J. R., Anders, C., Kivlighan, D. M., & Belcher Platt, A. A. (2021). Cultural ruptures: Addressing microaggressions in group therapy. *Group Dynamics: Theory, Research, and Practice*, *25*(1), 74–88. https://doi.org/10.1037/gdn0000149.

Moran, M. (2021). Resident/fellow census offers snapshot of trainee demographics. *Psychiatric News*. https://doi.org/10.1176/appi.pn.2021.2.20.

Munich, R. L. (1993). Varieties of learning in an experiential group. *International Journal of Group Psychotherapy*, *43*(3), 345–361. https://doi.org/10.1080/00207284.1993.11732598.

Ojo, E. & Hairston, D. (2021). Recruiting underrepresented minority students into psychiatry residency: A virtual diversity initiative. *Academic Psychiatry*, *45*(4), 440–444. https://doi.org/10.1007/s40596-021-01447-6.

Osseo-Asare, A., Balasuriya, L., Huot, S. J., Keene, D., Berg, D., Nunez-Smith, M., Genao, I., Latimore, D., & Boatright, D. (2018). Minority resident physicians' views on the role of race/ethnicity in their training experiences in the workplace. *JAMA Network Open*, *1*(5), e182723. https://doi.org/10.1001/jamanetworkopen.2018.2723.

Passel, J. S. (2008, February 11). U.S. population projections: 2005–2050. *Pew Research Center's Hispanic Trends Project*. www.pewresearch.org/hispanic/2008/02/11/us-population-projections-2005-2050.

Pepper, R. (2007). Too close for comfort: The impact of dual relationships on group therapy and group therapy training. *International Journal of Group Psychotherapy*, *57*(1), 13–59. https://doi.org/10.1521/ijgp.2007.57.1.13.

Popa-Velea, O., Trutescu, C.-I., & Diaconescu, L. V. (2019). The impact of Balint work on alexithymia, perceived stress, perceived social support and burnout among physicians working in palliative care: A longitudinal study. *International Journal of Occupational Medicine and Environmental Health*, *32*(1), 53–63. https://doi.org/10.13075/ijomeh.1896.01302.

Psychiatry Milestones The Accreditation Council for Graduate Medical Education. (2020). www.acgme.org/globalassets/pdfs/milestones/psychiatrymilestones.pdf.

Ribeiro, M. D. (Ed.). (2020). *Examining social identities and diversity issues in group therapy: Knocking at the boundaries*. Routledge/Taylor & Francis Group.

Rohrbaugh, R. M. & DeJong, S. M. (2022). The role of the program director in supporting diversity, equity, and inclusion. *Academic Psychiatry, 46*(2), 264–268. https://doi.org/10.1007/s40596-021-01474-3.

Sayrs, J. H. R. & Linehan, M. M. (2019). *DBT teams: Development and practice*. Guilford Press.

Shumaker, O., Ortiz, C., & Brenninkmeyer, L. (2011). Revisiting experiential group training in counselor education: A survey of master's-level programs. *The Journal for Specialists in Group Work, 36*(2), 111–128. https://doi.org/10.1080/01933922.2011.562742.

Snowden, L. R. (2003). Bias in mental health assessment and intervention: Theory and evidence. *American Journal of Public Health, 93*(2), 239–243. https://doi.org/10.2105/ajph.93.2.239.

Stay, F. A. W. I. (2020). Why I stay -The other side of underrepresentation in academia. *New England Journal of Medicine, 383*(4). https://doi.org/10.1056/NEJMpv2022100.

Stewart, A. J. (2021). Dismantling structural racism in academic psychiatry to achieve workforce diversity. *American Journal of Psychiatry, 178*(3), 210–212. https://doi.org/10.1176/appi.ajp.2020.21010025.

Sudak, D. M., Beck, J. S., & Wright, J. (2003). Cognitive behavioral therapy: A blueprint for attaining and assessing psychiatry resident competency. *Academic Psychiatry: The Journal of the American Association of Directors of Psychiatric Residency Training and the Association for Academic Psychiatry, 27*(3), 154–159. https://doi.org/10.1176/appi.ap.27.3.154.

Sudak, D. M. & Goldberg, D. A. (2012). Trends in psychotherapy training: A national survey of psychiatry residency training. *Academic Psychiatry: The Journal of the American Association of Directors of Psychiatric Residency Training and the Association for Academic Psychiatry, 36*(5), 369–373. https://doi.org/10.1176/appi.ap.11030057.

Sudak, D. M. & Stewart, A. J. (2021). Can we talk? The role of organized psychiatry in addressing structural racism to achieve diversity and inclusion in psychiatric workforce development. *Academic Psychiatry: The Journal of the American Association of Directors of Psychiatric Residency Training and the Association for Academic Psychiatry, 45*(1), 89–92. https://doi.org/10.1007/s40596-020-01393-9.

Sunderji, N., Malat, J., & Leszcz, M. (2013). Group day: Experiential learning about group psychotherapy for psychiatry residents at University of Toronto. *Academic Psychiatry, 37*(5), 352–354. https://doi.org/10.1176/appi.ap.12050096.

Swiller, H. I. (2011). Process groups. *International Journal of Group Psychotherapy, 61*(2), 262–273. https://doi.org/10.1521/ijgp.2011.61.2.262.

Tweedy, D. (2020, July 27). Opinion | Medical schools have historically been wrong on race. *The New York Times*. www.nytimes.com/2020/07/27/opinion/sunday/coronavirus-medicine-blackness.html.

U.S. Census Bureau. (n.d). *QuickFacts: United States*. Retrieved June 14, 2023, from www.census.gov/quickfacts/fact/table/US/IPE120221#qf-headnote-a.

Weinberg, H. (2023). Online training process groups for therapists: A proposed model. *International Journal of Group Psychotherapy, 73*(2), 141–165. https://doi.org/10.1080/00207284.2023.2170236.

White, K. (2002). *An introduction to the sociology of health and illness*. Sage Publications.

Willen, S. S. (2013). Confronting a "big huge gaping wound": Emotion and anxiety in a cultural sensitivity course for psychiatry residents. *Culture, Medicine and Psychiatry, 37*(2), 253–279. https://doi.org/10.1007/s11013-013-9310-6.

Willen, S. S. & Carpenter-Song, E. (2013). Cultural competence in action: "lifting the hood" on four case studies in medical education. *Culture, Medicine and Psychiatry, 37*(2), 241–252. https://doi.org/10.1007/s11013-013-9319-x.

Wyse, R., Hwang, W.-T., Ahmed, A. A., Richards, E., & Deville, C. (2020). Diversity by race, ethnicity, and sex within the US psychiatry physician workforce. *Academic Psychiatry: The Journal of the American Association of Directors of Psychiatric Residency Training and the Association for Academic Psychiatry, 44*(5), 523–530. https://doi.org/10.1007/s40596-020-01276-z.

Yardley, S., Teunissen, P. W., & Dornan, T. (2012). Experiential learning: Transforming theory into practice. *Medical Teacher, 34*(2), 161–164. https://doi.org/10.3109/0142159X.2012.643264.

Part II

Reflections on Diversity Dynamics

7 Rethinking the Group Leader's Interventions Addressing Diversity[1]

Haim Weinberg, with a response by Winston Gooden

Introduction

Although group therapy effectively contributes to the group members' well-being (Burlingame, 2021), it can also perpetuate existing power imbalances and reinforce dominant cultural norms, which can create barriers to treatment for marginalized individuals. Therefore, it is essential for group therapists to be aware of diversity dynamics in therapy. The awakening and intensifying of awareness in the U.S. and around the world about social injustice and discrimination against minoritized social subgroups in recent years has penetrated the boundaries of therapy groups and influenced their dynamics. Recently, social processes of divisiveness, splitting, and polarization quickly spread in the society-at-large, exposing conflicts and tension between social subgroups, increasing intolerance, and the loss of respectful dialogue. Many variations of these problematic dynamics are repeated in therapy groups, and it becomes very common to encounter hot conflicts about race and gender issues. Amid these confusing dilemmas, a lot of criticism is expressed from therapists who are keenly aware and sensitive to social injustice, stating that the common traditional interventions of group therapists are influenced by white supremacy or Eurocentric approaches and affected by theories composed by white scholars who did not pay enough attention to issues of diversity and equity. Some of these therapists (Gitterman, 2019; Ribeiro, 2020; Sue et al., 2019) suggested new ways of intervening in groups to address diversity, microaggressions, racial dynamics, etc.

All group therapists face the dilemma of how to relate to these issues:

1. How do we encourage a dialogue on these delicate topics?
2. How do we intervene in a way that will take into consideration all the sensitivities and vulnerabilities associated with racism, gender, and other power dynamics connected to a number of identities?
3. How do we avoid splitting and divisiveness in our therapy groups?

This chapter examines diversity dynamics in group therapy and explores the challenges that marginalized individuals face in accessing and participating in groups and the ways that group therapists deal with those challenges. It identifies some of the ways in which therapists work towards creating more inclusive therapeutic spaces, and how this differs from traditional group therapy. The chapter names the main differences between classical, traditional interventions used to address group dynamics, trauma, conflicts, and sub-grouping, and the new ideas that are expressed by colleagues who focus on

DOI: 10.4324/9781003455783-10

supporting BIPOC (Black, Indigenous, and People of Color) group members. In general, it identifies main dilemmas that distinguish between the old "white" schools of thought and the newer more inclusive perspectives. It points out two sets of mistakes that group leaders make: 1) ignoring diversity, racism, and microaggressions; and 2) responding to these issues in a rigid way. In addition, the chapter suggests some unconscious dynamics that might fuel those inclusive ideas when applied rigidly and to the extreme and tries to integrate the new and old approaches. Some group vignettes are presented in order to exemplify these ideas. The concluding response offers several suggestions in exploring this integration of classical and more inclusive approaches.

Conceptual Framework

Historical Context of Diversity in Therapy

Racism, discrimination, and other forms of injustice and mistreatment as a consequence of membership in marginalized groups, can result in trauma responses and chronic stress creating mental and physical health problems that negatively affect productivity and problem-solving (Hart, 2019). These populations may benefit from therapy, especially therapy that takes into consideration these trauma responses.

The history of therapy has been marked by a lack of diversity, with many early pioneers of psychotherapy coming from privileged backgrounds. For example, Sigmund Freud, the father of psychoanalysis, was a white, middle-class Austrian male, whose theories were based on his own experiences and cultural context. Freud's focus on the individual psyche and his disregard for social context and cultural factors in shaping psychological development has been criticized for reinforcing dominant cultural norms and perpetuating existing power imbalances (Chodorow, 1994; Weinstein, 2001).

In the 1960s and 1970s the civil rights movement and feminist movements in the United States brought attention to the lack of diversity in mental health treatment and called for more inclusive approaches. This led to the emergence of cultural and feminist psychology, which aimed to incorporate cultural and social factors into psychological theory and practice. In 1996, the book *Women and Group Psychotherapy*, edited by DeChant, dissected group therapy schools of thought one by one, showing how biased they were about gender. Since the feminist approach sees the source of personal problems as residing outside the individual but instead in society, feminist scholars criticized most group therapy approaches. However, despite these efforts, therapy continued to be dominated by white, middle-class practitioners, and in practice (and also most research) largely ignored the experiences of marginalized individuals. For example, in 2023 DeBlaere et al. found that 89 percent of the patients in their black female sample reported at least one instance of a racial microaggression by their therapist and, 43 percent reported some form of gender microaggression.

Challenges Faced by Marginalized Individuals in Group Therapy

Marginalized individuals face numerous challenges in accessing and participating in therapy, including stigma, discrimination, and lack of access to culturally responsive services. Subtle forms of discrimination can target any minoritized identity: gender, sexual orientation, religion, physical ability and learning differences, socioeconomic status, age, etc. (Nadal et al., 2010; Sue, 2010). For example, members of the LGBTQ+ community may be hesitant to seek therapy, owing to fear of discrimination, being pathologized, or simply a lack of understanding from therapists. Individuals from ethnic and racial minoritized groups may experience microaggressions (explained below), stereotyping, or culturally insensitive treatment from therapists. These experiences can lead to mistrust of mental health professionals, lack of engagement in therapy, avoidance of any kind of mental health treatment, and negative outcomes.

Miles et al. (2021) point out that whereas the occurrence and impact of microaggressions are well documented within individual psychotherapy literature, there is a paucity of research on the implications of microaggressions in group therapy. However, it is clear that marginalized individuals face additional challenges in group psychotherapy, where power dynamics and social hierarchies can become amplified. In groups, they are in even more danger of being misunderstood, stereotyped, labeled, and exposed to microaggressive comments from both the therapist and group members, since the group is a microcosm, reflecting what is happening in the outside world. For example, in a group of predominantly white, middle-class individuals, a member from a marginalized group may feel isolated or unheard. They may also face pressure to conform to dominant cultural norms and values, which can limit their ability to express themselves fully. These dynamics can create barriers to treatment and exacerbate existing mental health issues.

Group Interventions

Creating Inclusive Therapeutic Spaces

To address the challenges faced by marginalized individuals in group therapy, mental health professionals must work towards creating more inclusive therapeutic spaces. Schmidt (2018) recommends how group leaders can expand their skills and confidence to address racial microaggressions as learning and healing opportunities when they occur within groups. This can be achieved through a range of strategies, including:

1. Education and training: Group therapists should receive education and training on diversity dynamics in therapy and the ways in which cultural factors affect group dynamics.
2. Culturally responsive practice: Therapists should strive to provide culturally responsive treatment by incorporating the cultural and social context of their clients into their therapeutic approach. This may involve adapting treatment strategies to meet the needs of specific cultural groups, such as utilizing culturally relevant language, and acknowledging the impact of historical trauma on mental health.
3. Addressing power dynamics: Therapists should be aware of the power dynamics that exist in therapy, particularly in group settings, and work to create a safe and inclusive space for all members. This may involve addressing microaggressions (Sue, 2010), challenging dominant cultural norms, and encouraging all members to participate equally, or increasing understanding of the meaning behind the differences in participation and vulnerability in members. Not addressing these issues causes ruptures that should be repaired. Marmarosh (2021) writes that "One of the more common types of ruptures that we see are related to microaggressions in group therapy" (p. 213).

Common Mistakes in Addressing Diversity, Racism, and Equity in Group Therapy

Although the above strategies might help in creating an inclusive safer group environment for marginalized social subgroups, it is important for mental health professionals to critically examine the approaches they use to address diversity, racism, and equity in psychotherapy, and especially in group therapy. By recognizing the limitations of current practices, mental health professionals can strive to create more inclusive and effective therapeutic spaces.

In general, there are two sets of mistakes that group therapists make when addressing these issues:

A. Ignoring, Minimizing, or Behaving Insensitively

1. **Superficial Approaches**

   Group therapists may adopt superficial approaches to diversity by merely acknowledging differences in race, ethnicity, and gender without addressing systemic issues that perpetuate discrimination and inequality. This approach may create the illusion of progress without leading to meaningful change in addressing power imbalances and systemic oppression.
2. **Lack of Cultural Humility**

   Group therapists may lack cultural humility, which involves recognizing one's own cultural biases and limitations and being open to learning from diverse perspectives. This approach requires ongoing self-reflection and a commitment to challenging one's own assumptions and biases (Dixon et al., 2022; Miles et al., 2021; Tervalon & Murray-García, 1998).
3. **Tokenism** (King et al., 2010)

   In group therapy, mental health professionals may add one or two members from marginalized groups to the group to demonstrate inclusivity without addressing the underlying issues that impact the participation of marginalized individuals in therapy. It can create an unbearable burden on this one member to contain all the projections and stereotypes of other group members.
4. **Over-reliance on Individual-level Interventions**

   Group therapists may focus on individual-level interventions to address mental health disparities, such as teaching coping skills or changing thought patterns, without addressing systemic issues that perpetuate mental health disparities (Carter & Forsyth, 2010).

B. Applying an Overly Rigid Approach to Addressing Issues of DEI (Diversity, Equity, and Inclusion)

This short group vignette to demonstrate this kind of mistake[2]:

In a long-term online group for therapists, a newcomer joined the group. She was originally from a Muslim country, but moved to the U.S. when she was in her 20's, assimilated to the North American culture and did not practice any religious tradition. In the group she was quiet and kept an observing position. The group members warmly welcomed her participation and invited her more than once to respond to the topics that were discussed in the group. She did respond positively to these invitations, but more on the intellectual level and without expressing her emotions. To help, the group leader suggested exploring the difficulties for her participation. She explained that she was a shy girl and that she was worried that she would say dumb things. The group leader wondered more than once whether there was also a cultural component in her quietness, explaining that since she came from a conservative Muslim culture, where women's opinions are considered less important, perhaps it still affects her. She did not think that this was her case. One of the group members noticed some strange expression on her face and asked her whether she was irritated with the group leader for assuming repeatedly that her cultural background played a role in her quietness. She acknowledged that she was annoyed by the group leader's assumption since she perceived herself as well-integrated into the local culture.

In this case, the group therapist rigidly applied a culturally sensitive approach to an individual case, without checking whether it fit well. The problem was that the therapist reduced her experience solely to that lens and did not allow for exploration or connection to various other aspects of her experience (see later in the paragraph about intersectionality) as to what made her find herself to be "shy" and fear "she would say dumb things." The attempt of the group leader to add the cultural component and to be sensitive to the possible impact of unconscious social processes, resulted in the member feeling misunderstood.

1. How Do We Work With Trauma?

Working with trauma is always a delicate matter, and in groups, we should be even more cautious to avoid re-traumatization of group members. The main challenge in working with traumatized patients in the group is to create a safe-enough space in which they can work through their traumatic experiences without feeling overwhelmed or using dissociation. The work involves cautious delicate steps in which we help members feel grounded and regulate their flooded emotional state, before touching the trauma. However, in my opinion, it is better to work through the traumatic experiences rather than avoid them (unless we exceed the level of tolerance of the group member), and not to establish a "too safe" group atmosphere that prevents these experiences from being elaborated. In fact, the group is always a "semi-safe space" (Berman, 2019). The task of the group leader is to create enough safety to discuss uncomfortable feelings and unsafe situations. For example, if someone feels unsafe when a conflict erupts in the group (usually as a result of traumatic memories of difficult conflicts in the family of origin), in most cases the group leader should not prevent or avoid conflicts in the group but help the traumatized person to deal with this discomfort and strengthen their ability to face it.

However, when it comes to social trauma, such as the experience of Black people following years of enslavement and 400 hundred years of discrimination, it seems as if the recommendation for safety means not having to face uncomfortable feelings. For example, some extreme supporters of this approach claim that BIPOC patients should join only groups composed of other BIPOC members, since any encounter between BIPOC with White people (who are usually the majority in most of the groups) create an unsafe environment for the BIPOC members, resulting in re-traumatization. If we adopt this extreme approach, the question is whether BIPOC patients learn to work through their social trauma in the here-and-now or avoid it. This attitude, if applied too rigidly, does not help in addressing the sequelae of social traumas (Neuner, 2023). It does not fit the goal of group therapy as creating change for the individual. There may be times when a stage model of group therapy (such as recommended for the treatment of trauma by Herman, 1997 and Weinberg et al., 2005) is necessary to facilitate enough safety for members to address their traumas before being in a group which more closely represents daily life. Also, we should keep in mind that affinity groups serve different purposes from heterogenous groups and bring different challenges and benefits. For example, many affinity groups are designed to offer support centered around similar identities or shared values.

2. How to Intervene when Microaggressions are Made in the Group?

Microaggressions are described as subtle forms of discrimination, **often unintentional and unconscious**, that transmit negative and denigrating messages to a person or group based on an identity that has been marginalized. Racial microaggressions are "subtle, stunning, often automatic, and non-verbal exchanges which are 'put downs' by offenders. The cumulative weight of their never-ending burden is the major ingredient in black and white interactions" (Pierce et al., 1977, p. 66). For our discussion, it is important to keep in mind that these comments are often unintentional and even unconscious.

Sue (2010) suggests that there are two types of unconscious microaggressions: micro-invalidations and micro-insults. Micro-invalidations are communications that are not intended to inflict harm, but exclude, negate, and quash the feelings and lived experience of a marginalized person and/or demean the person's racial heritage and are characterized by rudeness and insensitivity. Micro-insults are subtle snubs that may or may not be known to the perpetrator that express an insulting message. Unconscious microaggressions can be combinations of invalidations and insults (Schmidt, 2018).

3. Trust the Process?

In the past, common practice suggested that when a group member expresses insulting comments towards another member, it is better to let the group respond ("trust the process") and **only if the group fails to do so**, the group leader might step in and wonder why the group is ignoring what is happening. The reasoning is that as group leaders we do not want to encourage dependency and prefer that the group develops its own way to deal with interpersonal tensions (of course, there are times when group leaders may have to provide a different way of navigating an impasse, since members tend to default to the adaptive, socio-cultural norms, e.g., avoiding talking about race).

However, when it comes to microaggressions, the more current recommendation of the current best practice approach is for the group leader to be very active and step in immediately, pointing out the microaggressive comment, bringing to the attention of the group the nature of this comment, and working with the member who expressed it on their unintentional and unconscious racial attitude (Lefforge et al., 2020).

Stevens and Abernethy (2017) encourage group therapists to address implicit bias as well. This active role is encouraged because BIPOC people have learned that any protest against microaggression is likely to result in either more aggression or "white fragility" where the offender's shame becomes the focus of the group. The dilemma here is how the group leader can support the BIPOC members to advocate for and protect themselves or focus on how the group can advocate for and protect each other, without being under or overly protective.

4. Confusing Conscious with Unconscious Attitude

As defined above, microaggression is often the expression of automatic, unintentional, and unconscious attitudes or comments. The best response is to bring it to the attention of the offender and explore the origin of the comment. However, group therapists and members sometimes respond to microaggression as if it is a deliberate, conscious behavior, by criticizing and attacking the offender. This assumption of conscious intent can be harmful for those who microaggress.

The same mistake holds for the concept of White supremacy. It can be misunderstood as a conscious, deliberate discrimination against target groups by extreme racists. The truth is that many of us from more privileged identities have been implicitly or explicitly socialized to see members of certain social groups as inferior, and may be unaware of this distortion and our own privileges. (This is a systems-centered view of discrimination rather than an individualistic view). In therapy groups we aim to draw members' attention to behaviors and attitudes of which they are unaware. It is important to be mindful that members' consciousness and awareness of this racialized socialization can vary dramatically and leader's intervention should be adapted in response to this.

5. How are We Supposed to Learn About the "Other?"

Usually, in group therapy, we encourage members to share their experiences, especially in the here-and-now. We do not want group members to assume how the other is feeling or experiencing the situation, and when someone is hurt, we want them to feel safe and empowered enough to express their feelings. In mentalization-based therapy (Bateman & Fonagy, 2013) the goal is to own one's subjectivity and assumptions, rather than telling people to not have them, since as it was stated before, we cannot control consciously these implicit biases. The responsibility for "educating" the other about the inner state of a group member lies on the shoulders of that group member. However, it seems that when it comes to diversity issues, White people are expected "to educate themselves". White people are encouraged to go to workshops about racism, read articles and books about them, and educate themselves about BIPOC experiences and the historical and current contexts regarding sociocultural issues. Although this may feel like an added responsibility for White people, this is consistent with the added responsibility that People of Color have to function in multiple roles. This preparation creates improved opportunity for deeper and less stigmatizing engagement for all.

While self-education is very important, and surely White people are likely to be ignorant about the impact of centuries of enslavement and discrimination, avoiding asking BIPOC or other minoritized group members about their experience in the here-and-now might lead to dangerous stereotyping and prevent people from learning. A sensitive white group member can approach a black member by saying: "I've read that many Black people were told that they should not speak up in the presence of White people. I don't want to make a wrong assumption, but is this why it's difficult for you to speak up in my presence?"

6. Rupture and Repair: Words May Harm

The best way to deal with microaggressions and insensitive comments in groups is to apply the practice of rupture and repair (Eubanks et al, 2021): Acknowledge the mistake or microaggressive comment, apologize authentically for the mistake, take responsibility for it, and take actions to repair the damage. To encourage group members to be able to do so, the group therapist should cultivate a culture in which mistakes are perceived as inevitable, part of human nature, and shift the emphasis from the attempt to avoid mistakes (or even microaggressions) to becoming curious about why they happened and learn how to repair them (Tronick and Gold, 2020).

Group members might respond to certain words in a very reactive way, triggered by their social trauma. For example, women can react to a male who did not respect their setting verbal boundaries in the group (e.g., saying that they do not want to talk about some topic, and being pressured by a man to do so despite their objection) as if they experienced a physical assault. Group therapists might join this traumatized response and blame the insensitive person as if an assault really occurred in the group. While words can definitely cause harm, and insensitive comments should certainly be addressed, words are not actions and do not kill. There is weight and impact to words, however, giving the same weight to words and to actions creates the opposite result; instead of recruiting the people who used offending words to become curious about what is behind their verbal expression, it alienates them, making them defensive. When this happens to White men following micro-aggressive comments they have made towards Black people, a strong disproportional reaction can simply evoke "white fragility" (DiAngelo, 2018), resulting in zero learning from the experience.

7. Intersectionality

Individuals can face overlapping systems of oppression and discrimination. These systems are based on how different marginalized identities intersect for an individual (Crenshaw, 1991). Intersectionality explains why the salience of one identity can make it difficult for a person to identify microaggressions targeting other identities such as gender, sexuality, socioeconomic status, religion, ability, etc. (Balsam et al., 2011). Group therapists should recognize the complex ways in which multiple identities intersect to shape individuals' experiences in therapy. This includes understanding the unique challenges faced by individuals who belong to multiple marginalized groups and how these experiences impact their mental health. For example, the American Psychological Association (2017) published guidelines for practice with Transgender and gender nonconforming people. The third guideline clarifies that gender identity and gender expression may have profound intersections with other aspects of identity.

Ignoring Intersectionality

Each of us has intersectional identities including age, ability, race, ethnicity, citizenship, nationality, sexual orientation, social class, gender, and many more aspects of ourselves. Mental health professionals may overlook the intersectionality of identities, which involves recognizing the ways in which multiple identities intersect to shape individuals' experiences in therapy. This approach may result in a failure to recognize the unique challenges faced by individuals who belong to multiple marginalized groups and how these experiences impact their mental health (Crenshaw, 1991). For example, the distressed reaction of many Black people to George Floyd's murder by the police, and their feeling that they are in a life-threatening situation every day, sometimes resulted in their belief that any mention of social injustice towards other minoritized groups was aimed to weaken the cry of "Black Lives Matter". Such a focus only on the issue of black racial identity to the exclusion of other marginalized identities can be viewed by some as ignoring intersectionality and other people's experience of marginalization. This does not mean that we should compare the suffering of different social subgroups. Comparing the suffering of anti-black racism to antisemitism to sexism to transphobia is ultimately unhelpful. Comparison leads to discrimination and discrimination leads to suffering (Thich Nhat Hanh, 2011).

In the group vignette mentioned at the beginning of this section (applying an overly rigid approach), the concern of the leader hyper focusing on one or two traits (female identity and Muslim background) may lead to ignoring other aspects of clients' experiences (e.g., autism, ADHD, ID, etc.) which could also be a factor of "being shy" and "thinking what I'll say will be dumb" from earlier.

A Group Vignette

A female member of a therapy group, 42 years-old, was usually passive, not speaking too much, but responsive to questions. She was from a traditional Chinese family who immigrated to the U.S., with a family that included her and two older brothers. When asked about her silence she explained that in her culture she is not supposed to express herself and her brothers were supposed to speak for her. Another group member, John, a white male, became quite irritated with this explanation, and said: "stop using your culture to make excuses for your helplessness! I know of many other Chinese women who have a strong voice". The group leader noticed that another woman in the group, Leona, who was originally from a Mexican family, was shrinking and had a strong emotional response. The group leader asked her whether she could verbalize her emotions, and she shared how distressed and unsafe she felt under John's attack, and that she was considering leaving the group. The group leader turned to John and asked for his response, but he couldn't understand what the fuss was about. The group leader tried to explain that his comment is considered microaggressive, but John dismissed it. Concerned about the impact of John's attitude on group members and being strongly influenced by the recommendation to step in actively when a microaggression comment is made in a group, the group leader criticized John for being unaware of his racist behavior, which only increased the conflict and tension in the group.

In a supervision session afterwards, the group leader understood that instead of exploring the reasons for John's comment, he took sides and probably made John feel attacked and unsafe as well. At the next group meeting he opened the group by apologizing for his mistake and working on repairing the rupture. It took several weeks to work through this event, explore its impact on group members, and restore the safe atmosphere in the group.

In this vignette the group leader applied the idea of actively dealing with microaggression too rigidly. Influenced by the idea that the group therapist should step in strongly when racism is expressed in the group, and fearing that group members might leave, he criticized and shamed John. If he was not triggered by John's comments, he might have instead taken the option of checking with the group members how they felt about John's comments or becoming curious what's behind John's inability to see how he hurt other group members.

Possible Hidden Dynamics

Perhaps the main dilemma that I point out in this chapter is whether group therapists focus on helping their group members to heal and have a better life, or whether their goal is beyond helping the specific group member or the group-as-a-whole. Group therapists might have a mission (sometimes hidden consciously or unconsciously) to heal society and to incorporate a social justice framework that "goes beyond raising awareness and addresses issues of equity, power relations, and institutionalized oppression" (Goodman, 2001, p. 5). These dynamics might be the hidden driving force behind this change in traditional group therapy. It is worthwhile to consider when our treatment groups are the best place to work towards healing society's ills and when we need to separate these two parts of our agendas to serve our patients most effectively. Perhaps an ethical approach is to be clear and inform the client regarding the goals of the group. Although this separation of interpersonal goals from broader societal goals is a common traditional stance, group therapy in its origins has included a consideration of the group as a social microcosm. Current ethics include a consideration of the continuity between the healing work within and between individuals and how this informs broader societal contexts. Groups provide a rich opportunity to work on multiple levels, preparation for this important group work is important as noted in Brabender and MacNair-Semands (2022).

Ethical Implications

This article is based on the following ethical imperative: "Group psychotherapists have an ethical obligation to adhere to the principle of Justice, ensuring that their groups serve all individuals" (Brabender & MacNair-Semands, 2022, p. 49). Multicultural competence requires that the group therapist acquires knowledge of how member's identities influence the individual experience and behavior. In their book, *The Ethics of Group Psychotherapy*, Brabender & MacNair-Semands (2022) go beyond the need to think about a group member's marginalized status, but also to be aware of and open to learning about the history, beliefs, values, and norms associated with the identities represented in the group.

The challenge in applying this ethical imperative in real group situations is that the way in which the group therapist is supposed to intervene in order to achieve it is a matter of interpretation. Some group therapists interpret it as protecting BIPOC from any psychological harm to the extent that group members who belong to the majority social group might feel too restricted in their ability to express themselves, although this goes against what the literature recommends. A way to frame this could be that suffering is universal and inevitable in some form. The goal may be to create meaning from the suffering occurring in a moment within the group. In fact, this dilemma exists in society-at-large, when people interpret the freedom of speech as freedom to express hurtful racist ideas. It is probably left for the group therapist to consider the complex ethical decisions in each case, beyond the ethical guidelines. However, being aware of the possible mistakes, both those of ignoring and of applying rigid interventions, can help the therapist to reach better decisions.

Limitations of the Existing Literature

While there has been increasing attention to diversity dynamics in therapy in recent years, there are still limitations to the existing literature. Many studies focus on the experiences of specific marginalized groups, such as individuals from ethnic and racial minority groups or LGBTQ+ individuals but fail to address the intersectionality of identities. Additionally, there is limited research on the experiences of individuals with different abilities, older adults, and individuals from low-income backgrounds in therapy.

Although there is evidence to suggest that culturally responsive therapy can be effective in improving mental health outcomes for marginalized individuals (Kirmayer & Jarvis, 2019), more research is needed to determine the most effective strategies for providing culturally responsive treatment.

Conclusion

The first part of this chapter sheds light on the critical importance of understanding and addressing diversity dynamics in group psychotherapy. While group therapy is an effective tool for promoting well-being, it can also inadvertently perpetuate power imbalances and exclude marginalized individuals. The increasing global awareness of social injustice and discrimination has inevitably influenced the dynamics of therapy groups, necessitating a thoughtful examination of how therapists engage with issues of race, gender, and equity. Recognizing the limitations of traditional approaches, this chapter explores the emerging ideas and interventions put forth by therapists who are committed to supporting BIPOC individuals and creating inclusive spaces. By identifying common mistakes, such as ignoring diversity and responding rigidly to these issues, the chapter encourages a nuanced and sensitive approach that considers the complexities of racism, microaggressions, and power dynamics. Additionally, it emphasizes the need for ongoing research in this area to inform best practices. Ultimately, by integrating new perspectives while building upon the foundations of classical group therapy, therapists can navigate the dilemmas posed by diversity dynamics, foster respectful dialogue, and create transformative therapeutic experiences for all group members.

Response by Winston Gooden

Weinberg rightly asserts that group psychotherapy offers a vehicle and processes that can address the often lack of availability of psychotherapy for persons from marginalized and minoritized communities. The group therapist will therefore need to go beyond attending to interpersonal issues, power dynamics, and group-level conflicts that are typically the focus of work in psychotherapy groups; the leader will need to find ways to address experiences of racism, marginalization, prejudice, discrimination, and other patterns of injustice that these clients bring to the group from their experiences in the majority culture, and will likely re-experience in the therapy group itself. The chapter therefore seeks to explore and address how the dynamics that diversity introduces into the therapy group can be acknowledged and addressed as an ongoing part of the group's therapeutic process.

One advantage of group therapy in handling the tasks of an ethnically and culturally heterogeneously composed group is that members, acting from their diverse ethnic, gender, sexual, religious identities and experiences, and so on, will create in the group a microcosm of the wider world consistent with experiences and expectations of social injustices and begin to display attitudes and expectations based on experiences from those worlds. When members recreate assumptions and take on roles similar to what they do in the outside world, the stage is set for experiences of hurt, pain, and misunderstandings within the group based on here and now perceptions of discrimination, slights, microaggressions, and bias, as well opportunities for insight, resolution, and repair. It is Weinberg's contention that groups so composed provide excellent opportunities for "Black, Indigenous, People of Color (BIPOC)" to access scarce yet much needed mental health services.

Leaders of these groups must pay careful attention to their personal preparation to lead such groups—taking advantage of educational experiences to deepen self-knowledge and understanding of discrimination, bias, racism and their impact on potential group members. The group therapist should be aware that groups may resurface painful memories and powerful emotions for certain members yet not for others, and be prepared to address the incidents and dynamics in the group that create a sense of unsafety for those at risk. Empathic understanding by the therapist of personal and vicarious experiences of marginalization and racist attacks, with its mixtures of shame, guilt, defensiveness, and anger, are likely to be present implicitly and explicitly. When these issues are alive in a group, empathic understanding by the therapist and a sense among impacted members that they are not carrying the burden alone because others are present who have similar experiences, are among the factors that determine a sense of safety. Thus, ensuring that a sufficient number of members from diverse backgrounds are part of the therapy group and that the leader is skilled at attending effectively to diversity dynamics as they occur, are especially important.

While the group process creates a rich context for learning and growth, its complexity is magnified by the intersection of various sub-identities of members. Weinberg makes a special point of the need to attend to intersectionality of gender, race, socio-economic status, religion, sexual orientation, etc. Attempts at addressing a salient area of identity may seem to ignore others that are really crucial for particular members. Attention to various sub-identities and their interactive impact for members of the group needs to be explored and addressed. Luckily this exploration and deepened understanding is also at the core of each member's work and part of the promise of healing in groups; so the therapist does not carry it alone, but must choreograph a process that recruits the members' deep engagement with it beyond their pain and hurt toward growth.

Addressing Diversity Dynamics

Weinberg warns against ignoring, minimizing, or superficially addressing diversity dynamics. Such superficial treatment exposes what he calls a lack of cultural humility that ignores one's own biases and permits a dismissal of the cultural experiences of others. This point is well taken because it is difficult to see how one whose experiences are not taken seriously can experience healing in such a context; one would be expected to sense the lack of serious interest on the part of the therapist, blame self, or become angry at the disrespect. When diversity is not taken seriously, its themes will not be given serious attention as part of the dynamics of the group and focus may be placed disproportionately on individual issues and dynamics while attention to issues of group composition may be left unaddressed as well.

Weinberg seems to believe that those who embrace the importance of issues of diversity in groups may risk taking a "rigid" approach to addressing these issues. Such rigidity means that diversity is so overconsuming that other important themes, issues and tasks relevant to the life and proper functioning of the group are ignored. Focus on a racial insult or an invalidating comment may mean that other important aspects of the group member's identity may be ignored.

Work on the intersections of identity may be sacrificed in favor of focus on a singular, though salient, dimension of identity. Aligned with this error may be the feeling of the therapist, implicitly or explicitly, that a member should be protected from a bruising interchange with others in the group or soothed in the midst of his/her pain. Such attempts to protect may impede the work of exploring and healing the retraumatizing effect of the insult, exclude the offender from an understanding of the impact of his/her actions toward the hurt party, leave unexamined the feelings of other individual members and ignore group-level meanings of the event. Such an approach may enfeeble the group and heighten its dependence on the therapist. Yet, while this caution is an important one, the question of how to support a hurt member who is at risk for further trauma and is at risk for premature termination, especially if she is one of only a few "BIPOC" members in that group, requires further discussion. Weinberg prefers an approach that "trusts the process" rather than a confrontation of the offender or the group that colludes with him or her. Use of a self-reflective approach to help the offending member who uses a microaggression in the group should help him/her to become aware of the hurt and the possible ways in which this takes place in other arenas of his/her life. This processing may even lead to an apology to the offended person that may diffuse the intensity of the hurt and the anxiety in the group.

Although Weinberg's approach acknowledges that the processing is to involve the offender, the group and possible subgroups as well as the victim and lead to healing and change for all, the therapist must decide, based on her knowledge of the members, the stage of the group and the impact of the disparaging comment on the individuals involved and on various subgroups, where to intervene first and how to mitigate the anger of the victim. The member attacked and the subgroup of members who share a similar diverse background are likely to be most offended and to require immediate attention and processing of the incident. Although both the perpetrator and victim need to experience the care of the therapist and understand that healing of hurt and the corrective transformation of each group member is the goal of the group and one to which each member contributes. The therapist must still decide when and where to intervene and with whom. That decision signals to the group what is to be given priority and whom. Neither the shame and guilt potentially experienced by the corrected perpetuator nor the hurt re-experienced by the victim can be ignored but can and should be taken up into the work of the group as it progresses and clarified along with such issues of white fragility and the hidden rewards of subtle putdowns, invalidations, and insults. With this difficult work undertaken the group becomes more cohesive and safer place for all the members.

Weinberg warns about the possible confusion of addressing behaviors conceptualized as originating from unconscious attitudes as if they are conscious thoughts and intentions. Microaggressions that insult or invalidate may be examples of unconscious bias rather than resulting from consciously held racist beliefs and attitudes. He suggests that helping a member access the unconscious processes related to an aggressive comment is more productive than intervening as though the offending member knew the hurt that would be caused and intended it. Though this approach will help the offending group member, it is important to acknowledge that the recipient of the insult feels the hurt—intended or not—and so will all the members who share that sub-identity. They will perhaps think that the slight or insult was intended. Does the therapist acknowledge and process the hurt feelings and the hope for an apology or does the leader first work to explore the source of the unconscious bias? Granted, the source of the comment may not be clear but the impact is usually available for observation and if the disruption in the recipient is obvious, may that not be the proper starting point for an intervention? How does the therapist acknowledge the hurt (unconscious in intent or not), help the victim cope with the insult and attendant feelings while also increasing the perpetrator's awareness of his/her unconscious bias or other motives for the comment? Who/what gets priority?

Member Disclosure

Weinberg claims that some therapists object to requests to have members from minority groups share their stories and experiences so that majority members may learn. He objects to this posture on the basis that majority members are asked to understand their group colleagues but are not permitted to ask for their stories lest such rehearsals retraumatize or otherwise upset the minoritized members. Weinberg wonders how members can get to know one another's stories if some are prohibited from asking. He sees this as a protective move that disrupts learning in the group and protects the unwilling member from exploring openly while giving others an opportunity to empathize, learn and revise stereotypes. While it is true that members in therapy groups teach each other by disclosing relevant experiences that help others understand and empathize, it is important to discern the difference between a natural unfolding of sharing and disclosure that leads to mutual appreciation, understanding, and care and command performances that are done for the benefit of others with a risk or sense of being judged or disrobed before a group in a process that is not mutual and for the other's gaze. Minoritized individuals often feel that they are being asked to become experts on the experiences of other people who shared their identity, and to bare their souls to persons they do not know well so that their audience may learn and grow. Such requests, if accepted, may well have negative results for those who comply. The issue is not the sharing of personal stories so that one becomes known and is able to benefit from the group as one helps others to share and grow—that much is part of the character of therapy groups and their power to heal—the intimacy so generated breeds acceptance and healing. The problem is if the request is one-sided, it reinforces power differentials and may contribute to premature or improper disclosures. The process of disclosure should begin with ground rules about disclosing that gives members of the whole group an opportunity to meta-disclose about disclosing, explore what disclosure will potentially involve, express fears and hopes about the process and agree upon limits of disclosure and the freedom of each member to establish their own boundaries for reasons of safety and self-respect. These will not be permanent but will be changed only when the person is ready to do so. With safety established and members informed and empowered to manage when they share they will be able to understand when disclosure is needed—though it may be uncomfortable and how to initiate it for their own benefit and for the group's development.

In cautioning against the danger of over-active intrusion in the group process to correct microaggression or to protect minoritized members from demands that may stir anger, anxiety, and or re-traumatization, Weinberg reminds us that "words do not kill". His concern seems to be that harsh words or demands in a group may be taken as an attack analogous to a physical attack outside of the group. When these are made to seem equally dangerous and the therapist acts to end the attack it cuts off further exploration of what motivated the comment and what its meaning might be for the perpetrator, the person treated unkindly and the group as a whole. This silencing prevents the rupture and repair process that may lead to deeper understanding, apology, and strengthened relations in the group.

Weinberg's concern is that therapists are exchanging process and exploration for direct action to protect minoritized members and/or to create social change in members from majority cultures who may be prejudiced. In this way they will make societal change directly in the group instead of in the society at large. I do not know if Weinberg's assumption is correct but is it worth further exploration? Are therapy groups laboratories for societal change? Are the values practiced in group therapy able to create social change in society at large? Are the deep values of well-run groups—listening, exploration of one's experiences, motives, and impact on others—sources of social change as well as individual change? These may not be the right questions to ask but the relation between processes of individual healing and reconciliation sponsored by group approaches to therapy and wider inter-group relations in societies are worth asking. So too are questions about how our knowledge of diversity, inclusion, and equity are relevant to increased effectiveness in group therapy, healing, and interpersonal change. While Weinberg's interest is in preserving the curative power of group therapy and not diffusing its traditional sources of efficacy, we may also wonder how group therapy can address large group and cultural issues of division, oppression, subjugation, and injustice. Certainly, when these themes appear in groups they need to be addressed on the group level with the best available tools and techniques; but the broader question of the societal roots of the difficulties we meet in group therapy and the vestiges of social ills that play out in groups and in the society as a whole must engage our interest, our attention, and our practice as well.

Endnotes

1 I want to thank Dr. Martha Gilmore for help in editing this chapter.
2 All case vignettes were disguised for confidentiality. Permission was given from the relevant group members.

References

American Psychological Association. (2017). Guidelines for psychological practice with transgender and gender nonconforming people. *American Psychologist*, *72*(4), 386–400. http://dx.doi.org/10.1037/a0039906.

Balsam, K. F., Molina, Y., Beadnell, B., Simoni, J., & Walters, K. (2011). Measuring multiple minority stress: The LGBT people of color microaggressions scale. *Cultural Diversity and Ethnic Minority Psychology*, *17*(2), 163–174. https://doi.org/10.1037/a0023244.

Bateman, A. & Fonagy, P. (2013). Mentalization-Based treatment. *Psychoanalytic Inquiry*, *33*, 595–613. https://doi.org/10.1080/07351690.2013.835170.

Berman, A. (2019). Therapeutic semi-safe space in group analysis. *Group Analysis, 52*(2), 190–203. https://doi.org/10.1177/0533316418815029.

Brabender, V. & MacNair-Semands, R. (2022). *The ethics of group psychotherapy: Principles and practical Strategies*. Routledge.

Burlingame, G. M., & Strauss, B., & Joyce, A. (2021). Efficacy of small group treatments: Foundation for evidence-based practice. In M. Barkham, W. Lutz, & L.G. Castonguay (Eds), *Bergin and Garfield's handbook of psychotherapy and behavior change: 50th anniversary edition* (pp. 583–624). John Wiley & Sons.

Carter, R. T. & Forsyth, J. (2010). Reactions to racial discrimination: Emotional stress and help-seeking behaviors. *Psychological Trauma: Theory, Research, Practice, and Policy, 2*(3), 183–191. https://doi.org/10.1037/a0020102.

Chodorow, N. J. (1994). *Femininities, masculinities, sexualities: Freud and beyond*. University Press of Kentucky.

Crenshaw, K. W. (1991). Mapping the margins: Intersectionality, identity politics, and violence against women of color. *Stanford Law Review, 43*(6), 1241–1299. http://dx.doi.org/10.2307/1229039.

DeBlaere, C., Zelaya, D. G., Dean, J.-A. B., Chadwick, C. N., Davis, D. E., Hook, J. N., & Owen, J. (2023). Multiple microaggressions and therapy outcomes: The indirect effects of cultural humility and working alliance with Black, Indigenous, women of color clients. *Professional Psychology: Research and Practice, 54*(2), 115–124. https://doi.org/10.1037/pro0000497.

DeChant, B. (1996). *Women and group psychotherapy*. Guilford Press.

DiAngelo, R. (2018). *White fragility: Why it's so hard for white people to talk about racism*. Beacon Press.

Dixon, K. M., Kivlighan, D. M., Jr., Hill, C. E., & Gelso, C. J. (2022). Cultural humility, working alliance, and Outcome Rating Scale in psychodynamic psychotherapy: Between-therapist, within-therapist, and within-client effects. *Journal of Counseling Psychology, 69*(3), 276–286. https://doi.org/10.1037/cou0000590.

Eubanks, C.F., Warren, J.T., & Muran J.C. (2021). Identifying ruptures and repairs in alliance-focused training group supervision. *International Journal of Group Psychotherapy, 71*(2), 275–309. https://doi.org/10.1080/00207284.2020.1805618.

Gitterman, P. (2019). Social identities, power, and privilege: The importance of difference in establishing early group cohesion. *International Journal of Group Psychotherapy, 69*(1), 99–125. https://doi.org/10.1080/00207284.2018.1484665https://doi.org/10.1080/00207284.2018.1484665.

Goodman, D.J. (2001). *Promoting diversity and social justice: Educating people from privileged groups*. Sage Publications.

Hanh, Thich Nhat (2011). *Reconciliation: Healing the inner child*. Parallax.

Hart, A. (2019). The Discriminatory gesture: A psychoanalytic consideration of posttraumatic reactions to incidents of racial discrimination. *Psychoanalytic Social Work, 26*(1), 5–24. https://doi.org/10.1080/15228878.2019.1604241.

Herman, J. L. (1997) *Trauma and recovery* (revised edition). Basic Books.

King, E. B., Hebl, M. R., George, J. M., & Matusik, S. F. (2010). Understanding tokenism: Antecedents and consequences of a psychological climate of gender inequity. *Journal of Management, 36*(2), 482–510. https://doi.org/10.1177/0149206308328508.

Kirmayer, L. J. & Jarvis, G. E. (2019). Culturally responsive services as a path to equity in mental healthcare. *Healthcare Papers, 18*(2), 11–23. https://doi.org/10.12927/hcpap.2019.25925.

Lefforge, N. L., Mclaughlin, S., Goates-Jones, M., & Mejia, C. (2020) A training model for addressing microaggressions in group psychotherapy. *International Journal of Group Psychotherapy, 70*(1), 128. https://doi.org/10.1080/00207284.2019.1680989.

Marmarosh, C. L. (2021). Ruptures and repairs in group psychotherapy: From theory to practice, *International Journal of Group Psychotherapy, 71*(2), 205–223. https://doi.org/10.1080/00207284.2020.1855893

Miles, J. R., Anders, C., Kivlighan, D. M. III, & Belcher Platt, A. A. (2021). Cultural ruptures: Addressing microaggressions in group therapy. *Group Dynamics: Theory, Research, and Practice, 25*(1), 74–88. https://doi.org/10.1037/gdn0000149

Nadal, K. L., Issa, M.-A., Griffin, K. E., Hamit, S., & Lyons, O. B. (2010). Religious microaggressions in the United States: Mental health implications for religious minority groups. In D. W. Sue (Ed.), *Microaggressions and marginality: Manifestation, dynamics, and impact* (pp. 287–310). John Wiley & Sons.

Neuner, F. (2023). Physical and social trauma: Towards an integrative transdiagnostic perspective on psychological trauma that involves threats to status and belonging, *Clinical Psychology Review, 99*, 102219, https://doi.org/10.1016/j.cpr.2022.102219.

Pierce, C., Carew, J., Pierce-Gonzalez, D., & Willis, D. (1977). An experiment in racism: TV commercials. *Education and Urban Society, 10*(1), 61–87. https://doi.org/10.1177/00131245770100.

Ribeiro, M. D. (2020). Intersectionality, social identities, and groups examined. In M.D. Ribeiro (Ed.), *Examining Social Identities and Diversity Issues in Group Therapy: Knocking at the Boundaries*, pp. 3–23. New York: Routledge.

Schmidt, C. (2018). Anatomy of racial micro-aggressions, *International Journal of Group Psychotherapy, 68*(4), 585–607. https://doi.org/10.1080/00207284.2017.1421469.

Stevens, F. & Abernethy, A. (2017). Neuroscience and racism: The power of groups for overcoming implicit bias. *International Journal of Group Psychotherapy, 24*(1), 1–24. https://doi.org/10.1080/00207284.2017.1315583.

Sue, D. W. (2010). *Microaggressions in everyday life: Race, gender, and sexual orientation*. Wiley.

Sue, D. W., Alsaidi, S., Awad, M. N., Glaeser, E., Calle, C. Z., & Mendez, N. (2019). Disarming racial microaggressions: Microintervention strategies for targets, White allies, and bystanders. *American Psychologist, 74*(1), 128–142. https://doi.org/10.1037/amp0000296.

Tervalon, M. & Murray-García, J. (1998). Cultural humility versus cultural competence: A critical distinction in defining physician training outcomes in multicultural education. *Journal of Health Care for the Poor and Underserved, 9*(2), 117–125. https://doi.org/10.1353/hpu.2010.0233.

Tronick, E. & Gold, C.M. (2020). *The power of discord*. Little, Brown Spark.

Weinberg H., Nuttman-Shwartz O., & Gilmore, M. (2005). Trauma groups: An overview. *Group Analysis, 38*(2), 189–204. https://doi.org/10.1177/05333164050523

Weinstein, F. (2001). *Freud, psychoanalysis, social theory: The unfulfilled promise*. State University of New York Press.

8 The Work of Overcoming Racism/White Supremacy in Group Therapy

Ron Hopson

Introduction

I argue in this chapter that racism/white supremacy is a predominant social and cultural ideology, and set of practices, which invades/impacts/influences the therapeutic environment of the psychotherapy group. Racism/white supremacy is a defining context in our lives as therapists, and the lives of our patients—of all races—and must be reckoned with in the clinical encounter. Recognition of this reality is crucial to the work of diversity. Recognition of this reality is crucial to therapeutic success, and training students of group psychotherapy to work with racism/white supremacy should be considered a necessary element of cultural competence.

Utilizing the work of Wilfred Bion, Ernest Becker, and others, I offer here a perspective on working with racism/white supremacy in group psychotherapy. I suggest there are four challenges which, if met, will aid in overcoming racism/white supremacy: 1) denial; 2) impaired empathy (and the failure to think); 3) shame; and 4) the fear/denial of death. I will discuss each in turn and end with a word on the possibility for passion—if we can overcome racism/white supremacy. This chapter is an expansion and update to a plenary talk that I gave at the American Group Psychotherapy Association Connect meeting in 2023.

Conceptual Framework

Meanings and Definitions

Throughout the chapter, I will use the terms racism/white supremacy conjointly. I ask that you bear with, or suffer with, my use of these terms. The term white supremacy, particularly, may seem overreaching in characterizing the reality of race relations. Generally, the term white supremacy conjures scenes of robes, torches, and violence. Carol Anderson (2016) details how this narrowing of the meaning of white supremacy to the extreme cases was carefully curated in the 1960s to leave unexamined the broader systemic and barely noticed manifestations of racism/white supremacy.

However, I am not limiting the understanding of racism/white supremacy to extreme examples of violence and brutality. Rather, I understand racism/white supremacy as a pervasive ideological environment, keyed to skin color, which structures the mundane givens of everyday life, and informs norms, social and economic structures, and both extremes of social privilege and disadvantage. Racism is constituted by preference, prejudice, privilege, and power, especially institutional and structural power. As to the term "white supremacy," (or as Resmaa Menakem (2017) more accurately expresses, "White body supremacy"), in addition to the extreme examples, here I follow Mills (2022), and D'Angelo (2018), and use

DOI: 10.4324/9781003455783-11

the term "white supremacy" to "capture the all-encompassing centrality and assumed superiority of people defined and perceived as white, and the practices based on this assumption" (D'Angelo, 2018, p. 28). Cornel West (1982) argues "the structure of modern discourse in the West secretes white supremacy" (p. 48). White supremacy is the larger field, the existential, ideological, and indeed biological context out of which racism emerges; it is the invisible ether in which we, to borrow a Biblical phrase, 'live and move and have our being' (Acts 17:28).

Racism/white supremacy then is the figure/ground of the problem of "othering" in contemporary society. Racism, the figure, white supremacy is the ground.

Participation in racism/white supremacy is often independent of one's willingness or intentionality. To benefit from racism/white supremacy one need not be white, to be harmed by racism/white supremacy one need not be Black. Racism/white supremacy impacts all persons. Frantz Fanon (2021) has called white supremacy the governing fiction of our time. Racism is the implementation strategy of white supremacy; racism is the symptom caused by the virus of white supremacy. To extend the metaphor, the problem of "othering" creates the opportunity for infection with the virus of white supremacy from which racism is a predominant symptom. Addressing the symptoms is an important step in treating the virus.

Consider the following: the growth of segregation to levels similar to fifty years ago (Menendian et al., 2021) and the relentless and terrifying harassment and public lynching of Black men and women at the hands of civilians and law enforcement. Year after year, the death penalty imposed on Black bodies, without due process, for simply "being while Black"—Amadou Diallo at his front door, Trayvon Martin in his neighborhood, George Floyd in his car, Michael Brown walking down the street in his neighborhood, Breonna Taylor in her own bed, Tyree Nichols in his car, and horribly, the list goes on. And then there is the harassment that stops short of death—Harvard professor Henry Louis Gates stopped as he entered his own home, or Christian Cooper (Black NYC birder) harassed by a white woman who threatened to call the police and report an African-American man threatening her, the pervasive harassment, inequities, the lynching, and the recurring dehumanizing spectacles, (the police would not have beaten a dog the way they beat Tyree Nichols). And much more. This is the relentless social and cultural environment infected by racism/white supremacy, which must be named. It is the environment in which our group members, and ourselves live. Frederick Douglass (1852), in his Fourth of July speech to a slave-holding nation, said of the brutalities and inequities of his time, what may be said of the brutalities and inequities of our time: If these things were taken seriously, they would "disgrace a nation of savages." Yet, these things proceed apace, in America (and sadly in other parts of the world). Racism implements the particular form of "othering"—white supremacist ideology, and white supremacist ideology hampers our ability to see and end the devastating scourge of racism.

In regard to racism/white supremacy, the work for those involved in doing group therapy is three-fold: First, to believe that racism/white supremacy is a relevant factor in the group process in both same-race and mixed-race contexts, that race matters, when race is being explicitly discussed, as well as when other topics seemingly unrelated to race are under consideration. Second, to understand how the reality of racism/white supremacy shows up in the group, and third: to apply effective interventions to illuminate and intervene when racism/white supremacy is operative in the group. These three tasks will be our focus throughout the chapter.

As racism/white supremacy is a fundamental structuring principle of U.S. society, racism/white supremacy can operate even when the group is not racially diverse. Therefore, the problem of racism/white supremacy is unavoidable and must be understood and 'worked' within the group—whatever the demographic make-up of the group. Racism/white supremacy is operative in groups as the invisible standard or foil, and the paradigmatic self/other template by which groups navigate the challenge of establishing shared identity. ". . . whiteness is the universal standard "against which a patient of color is understood to be different" (Brickman, 2018, p. 198), and by extension, whiteness is the universal standard by which all, including those designated white, are measured.

Othering

Racism/white supremacy exploits a universal phenomenon, the challenge of living with others. I will use the verb "othering" to express the phenomena of difference becoming reified, essentialized, and demeaned. Racism/white supremacy is a prototypical "othering" phenomenon. The development of the capacity to perceive an "other" and to maintain a sense of boundedness between self and the world is fundamental and primary (Braten, 1993, cited in Billow (2003). Developmentally, one of the earliest tasks of the infant is the capacity to perceive and tolerate the difference between self and other (Mahler, 2000), the paradigmatic "other" being (m)other. Second-generation psychoanalytic theorists (e.g., Klein, 2002), presciently postulated the critical importance of the earliest phases of development and the vicissitudes of self/other differentiation for adult adjustment. Later research (e.g., Bowlby and Ainsworth) validated some of these early ideas, suggesting that interpersonal styles of relating to others may be traced to earliest experiences with significant others. The tasks of perceiving and tolerating difference continues as the child's world expands beyond family to school, playground, groups, and ultimately the society. The other poses a challenge. "Lacan specifies that the question at issue is a query "about" the Other, both a question asked of the Other by the subject—What am I?—and one dependent upon the subject's understanding of the Other's desire—What should I be for you?" (George, 2022, p. 241). Self and other identity is inextricably bound in the working out of identity. Work on intersectionality (Crenshaw, 1995; Duran, 2020) has demonstrated the power of othering to seize upon any occasion of difference and make it a problem. Integrating lessons from effectively addressing racism/white supremacy and adapting these insights to the particular types of othering, can enhance diversity efforts in other areas, and address the broader challenge of eliminating negative othering.

When differences are perceived as essential, defining, and potentially problematic, those who are different become cast as the "negative other." Othering involves processes of identification and internalization. Negative othering involves projection, projective identification, splitting, and envy. White supremacy provides the perfect ideological grounding for developing negative racialized othering. The dark "other" is different and cast as potentially a problem. Through projection, the dark "other" becomes the container for disowned aspects of the ideal white self, both feared and admired, loathed, and desired. The dark "other" becomes a negative self-object (see Kohut, 2009). Following Freud, we might say this tendency to negative othering results from "narcissism of a minor differences" becoming tyrannical. Skin color is the minor difference, potentiating tyranny. Developing Jacque Lacan's thought, George (2022) suggests "race . . . ever emerges to organize enjoyment, script the body, and structure group and personal identification . . . race is the "answer to the core question of human subjectivity . . . and is fundamentally intertwined in our American Symbolic (p. 241).

Dealing with different others is the first challenge of a group. Groups, upon coming together, inevitably use the raw material of the larger cultural norms as a starting point for self, other, and group identity. Group members import the roles assigned to them by the larger society based upon their demographic characteristics. An ongoing task of the group is to avoid difference degrading into negative othering. Failure to successfully work with difference can lead to fractionalization and conflict (Yalom & Leszcz, 2020) impairing the group's ability to function as a therapeutic group.

Racism/white supremacy impairs group functioning in multi-racial groups and in same-race groups. In multi-racial groups, group members are perceived and responded to along the lines of the racial typologies or stereotypes of the larger racist/white supremacist society. In same-race groups, racism/white supremacy can operate as embedded, taken-for-granted, racially coded norms and values. Such norms as the absence of race or racism as an issue in all white groups, embody the white supremacist idea that white is normative and only 'people of color' are 'raced' in this society (Roediger, 1991). Blackness is culturally inferior (and therefore economically less productive), and preferred values of rationality, dispassion, competence, self-efficacy, and an insistence upon order even in the presence of inequity are encoded white (Bobo, 2000, cited in Bonilla-Silva, 2006). When group members (or the leader), fail to adhere to the prevailing norms and values, they risk being marginalized or ostracized. If these norms and values are left unexamined, they construct a barrier to full personhood for group members who do not (or cannot, due to their race) meet the standards, group cohesion—a critical therapeutic factor, is hindered, and the work of the group is subverted.

Group Interventions

On Groups Working

The fundamental work of a therapy group is to allow and support group members to discover themselves in the group, and for the group to affirm the full personhood of its members and support group members 'living into' their authentic self (Rogers, 1961). This is a useful framing for engaging the problem of racism/white supremacy in groups. Racism/white supremacy, by definition, impairs this work. Wilfred Bion's understanding of "work" illuminates what is at stake in racist/white supremacist systems.

The initial task of group members is to "establish contact with the emotional life of the group in which he lives . . ." (Bion, 1959, p. 127). To accomplish this task, the group member endows the group with certain assumed characteristics, norms, and values, drawn from the larger society. Thereby, the initial group identity is formed. The group member then, must 'find him/herself' within this group identity—establishing that they possess the normative characteristics necessary for membership in the group. Similarly, they must perceive that others also possess these characteristics. To the extent that the self, or other persons, are different in a way that prevents their possessing these characteristics, those persons are alienated from full value and membership in the group, and participation in the group process.

An example may be the old claim that therapists prefer those who are YAVIS (young, attractive, verbal, intelligent, single; Schofield, 1986)—to which I would add, white (YAWVIS). Persons in the group who do not possess these characteristics may be considered less than adequate to best utilize the therapeutic situation. Here the intersectionality of othering is evident—othering by age, attractiveness (e.g., predominantly European physical features), as well as social class and education. When these normative characteristics are 'the price of the ticket' to belong in the group, one of the key curative factors in groups—universality

(Yalom & Leszcz, 2020), is prevented, the group is fractured, persons are ostracized (or self-ostracize—'I am not one of them'), and the work of the group is impaired.

Bion maintains, "A group is working, to the extent that it's attitude, it's "mental activity" permits the recognition of the capacities of all the individuals in the group to contribute to the task at hand, to co-operate in coming to solutions for the problems for which the individual group members have sought help" (Bion, 1959, p. 129). The mental activity of racism/white supremacy necessarily involves othering—separation from and diminishment of the one who is 'othered'—in this case, by race. Recognition of the capacity of the 'raced' individuals is prevented. Racism/White supremacy prevents recognition across race, of the capacities of all of the members of the group. As some are relegated to the margins, all of the capacity of group members is not seen, and all of the capacity of the group cannot be realized.

Bion outlined positions that prevent groups from working. He called these positions "Basic Assumptions." Bion's Basic Assumptions are Dependency, Pairing, and Fight/Flight. Basic Assumptions are mental attitudes that, when present in a group, sabotage the work of the group, and create division and conflict. Basic Assumptions operate as unexamined, taken-for-granted, often unconscious—basic assumptions—foundational beliefs born of distortions, anxieties, and socialization. Basic Assumptions become the lens through which group members are perceived and group interactions are understood. When groups are unable to work through the distortions and anxieties which underpin Basic Assumptions, or what Harry Stack Sullivan (1953) would call "disintegrating tendencies," the group is unable to work, and the threat of disintegration looms on the horizon.

The role of the other can be seen in the operation of the Basic Assumptions. In Dependency, idealization is transposed, the self becomes the other, bereft of identity or efficacy, seeking psychic merger or deep identification with the leader (therapist or some powerful other), the ubermensch perhaps, who is the supreme all-wise one. Deviation from the dictates of the leader leads to the ostracizing and othering of the offending parties. In Pairing, two members find such resonance with one another as to exclude others (often including the therapist) from relevance, effectively othering the entire group. Those different from the idealized pair, are the denigrated other. In fight/flight the group has met to fight something or to run away from it. It is prepared to do either. Fight/Flight can be the source of simmering conflict within groups or the source of a sense of malaise and lost vitality, which often signals a group's effort to 'keep away from one another' while in close proximity. Within or outside of the group, those who are different in some relevant way, are the dangerous or intolerable other.

To Bion's triad of Basic Assumptions, I want to add a another, Racism/White supremacy.

Racism/White supremacy "lives in the bodies of Americans" (Menakem, 2017) informing much of our living: "we humans are self-interpreting beings who at any time and place have a need to make sense of our experience and . . . This need to make sense of our condition commonly has recourse to a codified system of interpretation . . . which partakes of the biases and assumptions of the community that gives rise to it" (Brickman, 2018, p. 197). Given the formative nature of racism/white supremacy, fundamental to the founding of the U.S., I suggest racism/white supremacy be considered a root Basic Assumption in the U.S. context.

Racism/White supremacy may determine how other Basic Assumptions operate. As an example, in Dependence, group members look to the leader to determine what is to be done in the group. 'You are the experts, give us instructions, what are we supposed to talk about, how shall we help one another? However, if the therapist(s) are persons of color there may be rejection of the tendency to initially depend upon the group leader, leading to an enactment of resistance or opposition.

Case Example

I joined as therapist an ongoing therapy group, replacing a therapist who was perceived as being white, who had left the group temporarily for four months due to a family matter. The regular therapist shared the reason for her departure but the length of her absence was not initially known by the group. Early on, I encountered vigorous resistance particularly from one of the white members of the group (also a therapist). Often, when I made comments, interventions, or interpretations, she would immediately object, challenge, or refute my efforts. Beyond preventing her own access to therapeutic assistance, this behavior threatened to undermine the group as a whole. By the fourth group meeting the other group members were able to support my efforts to examine the challenging member's behavior and invite her introspection about the situation. The challenging group member had characteristically been very supportive of the prior therapist—'hanging on every word,' as one group member put it, demonstrating significant dependence upon the previous therapist's wise interventions. The challenge was to understand why the difference in her attitude toward me. As we worked with this question, the issue of race was put on the floor (by another group member). Her initial response was to disavow racist sentiment regarding my competence, and actively resist considering this possibility. This disavowal of racist feelings is a common manifestation of a vertical split. As we persisted in the investigation, we were able to uncover that this group member was deeply disappointed that a man, and a man of color had replaced the prior therapist. She feared I would be unable to provide the needed insight and containment that the prior therapist had provided and though initially hesitant to acknowledge it, wondered about my competence. Her dependency reflexes were thwarted by the gender bias and implicit racism/white supremacy of which she was unaware, and perhaps by professional envy or competitiveness.

In this case, Dependency was replaced with Fight/Flight as the challenging group member worked against her impulse toward dependency by rejecting any efforts by this person of color to assist her, or indeed other group members. I understood this as a defensive posture which could be explained by both the racial and gender differences between myself and the group member. We also attempted to work with the group member's shame around their implicit bias (working with shame will be discussed below).

Denial

The challenging patient's initial insistence that race was not an aspect of her response to me, as it later became evident that it was, is an example of denial. Others in the group also initially tried to deny racial bias as an element of the patient's response to me. This is to be expected when groups are confronted with racial issues. Denial is often a first reaction to considerations of racism. As with white supremacy, the term racism can land harshly and lead to an initial reaction of denial/disavowal. The seemingly small incidences of apparently racialized thinking or microaggressions, are allowed to pass unexamined and unchallenged. When only the grotesque events are considered racist, then racism/white supremacy can be seen as an aberration rather than the norm. We selectively ignore the mundane occasions of something "impolite" or literally off-color, microaggressions, the stubborn structural barriers and banal procedural impediments to equity which contribute to the atmosphere which makes the major outrages possible. We remain ignorant of, and innocent regarding the more pedestrian moments of racism/white supremacy. James Baldwin (1962/63), in his *Letter to My Nephew* said of this phenomena: "it is not permissible that the authors (or I might add: benefactors) of such devastation should also be innocent. It is the innocence which constitutes the crime" (p. 6). Toni Morrison called this denial/innocence—"willful oblivion," Scott Peck (1985) labeled the refusal to see the potential for injustice, disadvantage, or harm, "militant ignorance."

Harry Stack Sullivan's (1953) description of selective inattention well describes this tendency: "By selective inattention, we fail to recognize the actual import of a good many things we see, hear, think, do and say . . . because the process of inferential analysis is opposed by (the self-system)—our self-concept. Clear recognition of the implications of matters to which we are selectively inattentive would call for basic change, it would make us either more, or in some cases less, competent, but in any case, different from the way we now conceive ourself to be" (p. 217).

Denial around matters of racism/white supremacy manifests overtly when frank discriminatory or prejudiced words and actions, or microaggressions, are met with resistance or disavowal, when challenged. Denial manifests covertly when taken-for-granted perspectives assumed to be 'shared by all,' or 'just the way things are,' are not examined and, if necessary, challenged. Perhaps one of the more troubling covert manifestations of denial about racism/white supremacy is the insistence on color-blindness in the presence of stark evidence of racial segregation in almost all spheres of life: "whites do not interpret their hyper segregation from blacks as a problem because they do not interpret this as a racial phenomenon instead they normalize this crucial aspect of their lives by either not regarding it as an issue or interpreting it as normal as 'just the way things are'" (Bonilla-Silva, 2006, p. 113).

Impaired Empathy

Denial, the refusal to see the implications of racially tinged everyday realities, is evidence of the moral injury of racism/white supremacy. That moral injury is an impaired capacity for empathy, or capacity for concern for the racialized other. As Charles Blow has said: "One doesn't have to operate with great malice to do great harm. The absence of empathy and understanding are sufficient" (Cited in Menakem, 2017). Winnicott (1965) identified the capacity for concern as a crucial developmental achievement of the child, necessary for satisfying reciprocity in the interpersonal world. The capacity for concern is the necessary precondition to the development of empathy.

Baron-Cohen (2011) defines empathy in a manner that has particular relevance for group work. "Empathy occurs when we suspend our single-minded focus of attention, and instead adopt a double-minded focus of attention . . . (it is) our ability to identify what someone else is thinking or feeling, and to respond to their thoughts and feelings with an appropriate emotion" (pp. 10–11). The capacity to feel with and for, another, is a critical reparative and restorative function in group therapy. Yalom states: "What is important, though, is not only that early familial conflicts are relieved, but that they are relived correctively . . . For many patients, then, working out problems with therapists and other members is also working through unfinished business from long ago" (Yalom, 1970, p. 14).

For conflicts to be relived correctively, group members must be capable of and willing to identify what others are feeling and respond appropriately. The potential for healing and transformation occurs when group members are able to empathize with one another.

"Empathy erosion" (Baron-Cohen, 2011) happens when people are turned into objects. Objectification is the endpoint of "othering." Ideologies and ideas rooted in racism/white supremacy objectify the racial other who is not seen as possessing thoughts and feelings similar to the self. Objectification impairs empathy.

Impaired empathy of the majority population can be seen in the stubborn refusal by many to recognize the implications of the systemic racialized inequities in plain view (Menendian et al., 2021). These inequities impinge upon the life possibilities and well-being of all persons, not just persons of color. They are brought into the group in many ways including: unconsciousness of privilege, for "raced" group members—pervasive low-level depression, anxiety or anger from coping with the weight of racism/white supremacy, for non-raced group members—unconscious guilt about privilege or guilt about the failure to overcome structural inequities, counter-phobic tireless activism hoping to singlehandedly eliminate racial oppression, despair, etc. The work of the therapist, and indeed the work of the group, is to identify and name the roots of such phenomena, and work with the group and individual members, to understand the source, and support restoration of the capacity for empathy and understanding.

The restoration of empathy, the restoration of the capacity for concern, the capacity to see the "other" as fully human, is part of the work of the effective therapy group. This is the task for those "othering" as well as those who are "othered." All are vulnerable to the "empathy incapacitation" of racism/white supremacy, even individuals from the same racial group. The dehumanizing beating death of Tyree Nichols by African American police tragically illustrates this reality.

Supporting the development of empathy may involve the group therapist in a more active way within the group. Strategies may include: Inviting group members across differences to imagine being in the position of the "other" and articulate what that may be like; rearranging the seating in the group to place people in closer proximity to the "other;" interpreting the split within a group member: 'I wonder if a part of you resonates with what at the same time feels alien to you?' The effort here is to arouse in the group the nascent capacities for human connection across difference, which racism/white supremacy has obscured.

Empathy Through Thinking

The ability to know and respond appropriately to what others are feeling is the achievement of intersubjectivity which racism/white supremacy disallows: "Both an individual's isolation and his immersion in a crowd exclude intersubjectivity proper, the encounter with an other" (Zizek, 2008, p. 31). This work requires the capacity to think. Bion (1963) uses the term "thinking" in a technical sense to mean a "linking" or connecting activity. Thinking involves recognition and acceptance of reality; it involves tolerating emotional engagement, tolerating the emotional reality of an-other (Billow, 2003). To think, in regard to racism/white supremacy, is to bear the emotional awareness, the lived reality of the racialized other. To think in regard to racism/white supremacy is to recognize the reality of the impact of racism/white supremacy on white and non-white persons and to feel the appropriate emotions.

Earlier I asked you to "suffer" my use of the term white supremacy. I used the term "suffer" deliberately because thinking may involve suffering; it may involve psychic pain as previously denied aspects of reality are finally recognized. Groups attempt to evade pain by evading thinking. Rather than empathetically tolerating the pain of racism/white supremacy as it impacts oneself and others, and allowing the pain to transform intention, awaken attention and inform future action, the group may move to the various forms of denial and disavowal: a sudden incapacity to think, outrage, attempts to assuage the victim, ignoring the racial component of the offense and focusing elsewhere, or resorting to despair—e.g., 'nothing can be done about this intractable problem.' Groups tend to resist "thinking" in regards to racism/white supremacy. Instead of thinking, we engage in what Bion (1959) calls "synthetic animation." On matters of race we opt for performative comity, what Peck (1990) called "pseudo-community," rather than authentic connection based upon shared empathy and recognition of the capacities and value of the other. Groups enact a racial façade, a racial false self. "The person who bears to think and to learn, risks ever-greater separation from established conventional relations with others, as well as with one's previous ideas" (Billow, 2003). Thinking then makes possible greater separation from established conventional relations based upon racism/white supremacy as awareness of the "other" increases.

To achieve more than "synthetic animation," in order to think, the group must risk the messiness of confrontation with difference and endure what I will call "productive chaos." The confrontation with (racial) difference can initially invite resistance, frustration and expressions of feeling harassed by the topic or by the invitation to think regarding the racialized other: ". . . the other is just fine, but only insofar as his presence is not intrusive insofar as this other is not really other "(Zizek, 2008, p. 41), conformity to prevailing norms rather than authentic presence is required of the other. Productive chaos can be the space where multiple voices and perspectives, which had been previously marginalized, insist on being heard, acknowledged, and reckoned with as fully equal human beings (Black Lives Matter is an example of this). The therapist offers the challenge to engage difference with empathy rather than othering. Productive chaos is the period where the established order (within the group, or in the world outside of the group) is no longer presumed to be appropriate and inevitable. This is the space where the invitation to think is offered and the work of coming to an awareness of the full humanity and equality of the "other" becomes possible. Here the macroaggressions and microaggressions, though they may be unintentional, are named, and recognition of the implications of these actions and attitudes is tolerated. Denial, selective inattention, ignorance, innocence are challenged, and the possibility for fuller awareness of the reality of those previously designated "other," emerges. Thinking allows movement from a stance of unawareness or superficial cordiality, to more authenticity.

Achieving the capacity to think will require the group to endure a period of chaos. The challenge of the therapist is to recognize when the chaos is productive. Signs of productive chaos include: the group feeling more alive and more group members actively engaged and attentive, those on the margins of the group claiming space and voice, or being empathetically attended to by the larger group, changes in roles among group members, absence of palpable fear despite vigorous group exchanges, exchanges between group members that suggest greater authenticity. The task of the therapist is to 'hold' the group through the moments of chaos. This may be done through the therapist verbalizations to the group recognizing the different feel of group activity, articulating how the chaos is productive, encouraging the group to continue moving, assurance that the therapist is watchful to prevent injury to group members, and offering faith and hope that the changes in the group, and group members will be positive. The work of the therapist is to maintain confidence in the ability of the group to work through what is necessary for the group members to achieve fuller authentic personhood, and for the group as a whole to be a place of inclusion and belonging: "to take care of the group is the assignment of the therapist, then the group will take care of its members" (James Anthony cited in Grotjahn, 1977, p. 129).

Shame

As the group awakens to the fact of racism/white supremacy and develops empathy for the damage wrought by this root Basic Assumption, in society and in the group, the recovery of empathy may involve the emergence of shame. I do not mean here pathological shame resulting from trauma, or shame emerging from the triggering of unresolved identification with early rejecting figures. Rather, I mean shame born of empathy. Shame may be in evidence when invitations to think, regarding racism/white supremacy, are met with: 'this is uncomfortable, must we keep talking about this?' I didn't do it, no one I know owned slaves, that was then, this is now . . .,' ' we suffer too . . .' 'this only divides us, it doesn't bring us together . . .' These protestations can be seen as evidence of the desire to avoid the suffering which attends acceptance of our racial reality (Ruth King, 2018). However, shame is a valuable pro-social emotion when it can be metabolized, worked through, and utilized productively to provide information toward change in one's behavior, allegiances or identifications.

Shame which signals an unintended disruption in the interpersonal bridge (Kaufman, 1992), can mobilize the desire for restored human connection. This is a particularly powerful element of group therapy. If group members can bear to do the shame-work—acknowledge and work through shame, in close proximity to others, the need to continue to deny the pervasive reality of racism/white supremacy is lessened. Shame can be the signal of awakened empathy, and can prompt reexamination of the self, and the taken-for-granted. If group members can tolerate it, shame can prompt vigilance against participation in furthering racism/white supremacy. Shame can provide motivation to repair the breach between one's ideals and reality, and between one's self and the "other." Shame, when tolerated, can provide wisdom toward restoration and repair, and can prompt a shift from allegiance to norms and ideas which objectify and create the "other," to solidarity with the human family—a necessary step in overcoming racism/white supremacy (Van Bavel & Packer, 2021).

Working with shame in group, the group therapist is challenged to provide holding and tension regulation while facilitating engagement with the powerful feelings of shame. "Often group members cultural wounds, biases and defensive reactions have evoked relational discord and shame, and the group therapist needs to strike a delicate balance between maintaining group trust and safety and encouraging the addressing of sensitive and painful issues" (Kaklauskas & Nettles, 2020, p. 29). However, this cautionary note should not be taken as conveying hesitance to address these issues in group, the group is not fragile (Grotjahn, 1977). As group members confront their prejudices and implicit biases, the therapist must also guard against the desire to avoid or deny these troubling realities. The task is to balance holding—encouraging of further exploration even as tension increases, with tension regulation—helping the patient and group titrate the feelings of shame such that the feelings inform and empower action in a different direction, rather than self-attack and group ostracism. Naming the shame-work as it unfolds, and explaining the value of forward-looking shame to the group can also assist in productive work around the emergence of shame.

As shame is resolved, the group, and group members face the question; how to change. The stubborn tenacity of racism/white supremacy, despite the costs, suggests a powerful disincentive to change must be at play. Many have linked the power of racism/white supremacy to fundamental economic structures (e.g., Marable, 2015). Yet, the recent resurgence of racism/white supremacy may suggest something more fundamental than economics, which keeps the destructive othering ideology of racism/white supremacy in place. Perspectives on the dynamics of change in psychotherapy may be informative.

Fear/Denial of Death

Once shame is faced and the willingness to change is embraced, the specter of loss emerges. Important to the work of significant change is loss and mourning. The work in rooting out the United States' root Basic Assumption will involve mourning the loss of power, privilege, and position, confronting the death of the old familiar, well-ordered but unjust ways of being. The Bugentals' (1984) wonderfully illuminated the challenges of change in psychotherapy in their paper: "A fate worse than death: the fear of changing." Change can involve more than acquiring new emotional or behavioral habits. Abandoning Racism/White supremacy as a root Basic Assumption may involve losing aspects of what has come to define the person and structure their life. Change involves transformation at the intrapsychic, interpersonal, and social level. Change can mean loss of aspects of one's identity and identifications (both who I am, and with whom do I belong?). Coming to awareness of the impact of racism/white supremacy may involve shifts in our relationship to and understanding of important figures from earliest childhood. Change involves the willingness to loosen old ties and idealizations of significant others based upon denial and selective inattention. Long-standing identifications and internal representations may take on added dimensions (e.g., the kindly grandparent's previously overlooked stubborn bigotry becomes a part of the internal representation of the grandparent). Views of the self may also change as one becomes more aware of unconscious and implicit attitudes which do not align with personal ideals. Also, giving up racism/white supremacy may involve changes in important relationships, changes that threaten significant renegotiation, or even loss.

The sense of change as death is made stronger by how racism/white supremacy invites a sense of security within group identity. When the identity of the group is called into question (e.g., the supremacy of whiteness), the sense of "participation in omnipotence" (Becker, 1973, p. 123), the sense of security derived from the group is threatened. The loss of a sense of familiarity, continuity and a loss of accustomed signifiers of one's identity—the loss of the primary identificatory group, can feel like something akin to existential dread. The end of racism/white supremacy can portend something beyond death of the personal self, death of something larger, the societal way of being, and death of the group to which one belongs, and which gave one identity.

Consider the chants of the racists/white supremacists marching in Charlottesville, Virginia. "Jews will not replace us . . . you will not replace us" was the chant. We will not be replaced. This is racism/white supremacy in its starkest realization, the fear of death, and the denial of death; we fear you will replace us, we refuse to be replaced by some "other," we refuse to allow our system of racism/white supremacy, to die—no matter the cost. This fear of death/denial of death is the impetus behind the Great Replacement rhetoric, —'some alien other will replace us.' This existential dread, death fear, or perhaps more properly put, annihilation anxiety, is provoked by rhetoric about orderly (read: white) society being destroyed by the prototypical "other," the dark hordes roaming our streets, or invading from the south. The fear of death then is manipulated by racism/white supremacist appeals to threat and the promise of safety through "othering," (white) group solidarity, and readily available resort to violence.

The fear of death/fear of group annihilation is managed by embeddedness in a world of imagined infallibility . . ." the desire to keep oneself tucked into a larger source of power. It is these things that make for the mystique of "group," "nation," "blood," "mother- or fatherland" . . . they keep one in the prison of the motherly racial national religious fixation (Becker, p. 134). The illusion of immortality (Adler: collective eternity impulse) is maintained by this deep identification with the group (Freud: horde). Terror management research has demonstrated how the fear of death lies behind appeals to nationalism and how death fear is related to bias against persons perceived as outside one's group identity—the "other" becomes the scapegoat and "only scapegoats can relieve one of his own stark death fear" (Becker, p. 149). "It is easier to dispose of troublesome thoughts of death when one disparages "different" others" (Solomon, Greenberg & Pyszczynski, 2015, p. 132). The scapegoat/other is subject to indifference (lack of empathy), hostility, ostracism, or even violence—"the terrifying sadism of group activity" (Becker, p. 133). "One thing that never ceases to surprise the native ethical consciousness is how the very same people who commit terrible acts of violence towards their enemies can display warm humanity and gentle care for the members of their own group . . . Refusing the same basic ethical rights to those outside our community as to those inside it is something that does not come naturally to a human being. It is a violation of our spontaneous ethical proclivity. It involves brutal repression and denial" Zizek, 2008, p. 48).

The work of the therapist is to create conditions to lift the repression and denial and name the existential fear which underlies resistance to change. Though challenging, this work of the therapist may support development of the more natural "spontaneous ethical proclivity" of the group. As group members engage the possibility for change in regard to racism/white supremacy, the therapist has the opportunity to hold space for the group to titrate the feelings around the reality of loss and the fear of the unfamiliar new self (or society) which may be possible. Fear of extinction through relinquishing racial group identification is named and challenged, and alternative identificatory possibilities are offered (e.g., human solidarity rather than subgroup exclusivism).

The therapist and the group are invited to relinquish the taken-for-granted defining and structuring ideologies of racism/white supremacy, and the illusion of immortality, born of deep identification with a group. This is for Bion, an act of faith. Here Bion borrows from the best of religious tradition in regards to meeting uncertainty and death: "the discipline that I propose for the analyst, namely avoidance of memory and desire (avoiding memory of the omnipotence born of belonging to one's primary group, and desire for conformity to the primary group—at any cost), increases his ability to exercise acts of faith" (Bion, 1977, p. 34). To meet the fear of change as death, faith is the proper response (Eigen, 1985). The therapist must hold out faith for, and faith in, the group. That is, the therapist must hold faith for the group, that a way of being and a way of being together, which does not dehumanize, demean, and divide, is possible, even as the group struggles with productive chaos. And the therapist must hold faith in the group; the conviction that the group can work through what is needed to overcome racism/white supremacy—at least as it operates in the group and in the group member's lives. 'Acts of faith' for the therapist involve the willingness to inquire, name and intervene when the Racism/White supremacy Basic Assumption is suspected or in evidence in the group. This is not done by prescribing another way of being, but rather by supporting the exploration of discontent and shame, and the fear of death, which may be evident underneath the racist/white supremacist group dynamic. Acts of faith for the group, involve the willingness to begin to think (in Bion's technical sense discussed above) regarding racism/white supremacy, and bear the shame, anxiety and death fears which may emerge. Doing this work in a group context has great potential, even at the neurological level. Gantt (2020) quotes Badenoch and Cox (2010): "one of the strengths of group therapy is the high likelihood that the neural networks holding early implicit experience will be triggered . . . as other members bring their struggles into the group the group can become an empathy rich environment for holding the pain and fear that emerges . . . as both therapist and group members understand more about brain development they become more capable of seeing other members and themselves with understanding and compassion. Such attunement helps to repair the circuits of regulation not only for the receiver of care but for the giver of care as well" (p. 157).

Wake Work

Working with death anxiety involves disorientation, mourning, and then awakening, as the social environment and the self, previously established along racist/white supremacist lines, are revealed to be self and other limiting, and indeed destructive. Helen Morgan (2021) in a talk on her book *The Work of Whiteness: A Psychoanalytic Perspective* presented at the Tavistock Foundation (2021), utilizes the work of Cristina Sharpe (2016) and her call for "work" regarding racism/white supremacy. A wake of course is the track of water behind a boat as it moves. A wake is also the time of sitting with the body of the deceased, beginning the process of letting go, mourning and recognition of loss after a death. And to be a-wake—here I assert the positive meaning of the much-maligned word "woke"—to be woke, is to be conscious, to be aware of the reality of one's environment, to be willing to think, and feel regarding oneself and others.

Groups, as microcosms of family and society, are particularly well suited to do wake-work around racism/white supremacy. If this work can be done, the long wake (as in water trailing a boat) of racism/white supremacy can be ended and the wake as mourning, and morning (awakening), can begin. Wake work involves coming out of denial and acknowledging the implications for all, of the long wake of racism/white supremacy, naming the psychic, physical and social damage of white privilege and the moral injury to all, of the racist/white supremacist structures and systems. Wake work involves recognizing how racism/white supremacy is operating in the group and in group members, and tolerating the fear of death which emerges when this recognition leads to naming, working through, and the possibility of change. And wake work means doing the work of mourning the loss of the familiar sense of self, others, and society as change is embraced, and holding faith in what is possible.

Implications for Training and Practice

The therapist may address the reality of the long wake of racism/white supremacy by inviting the group to consider how race may be involved in the issues of the group, whether or not there is a "raced" ("diverse") person in the group. This invitation will usually be met with the question: "what does race have to do with X (the current subject)? In all white groups, this may be particularly challenging. In all groups, raising the issue of race may involve the therapist bearing attacks on the leader as the pain of awakening begins to be experienced and initially resisted. It is important that the therapist avoid colluding with denial by conceding to the group's resistance to awakening. If race is not an immediate factor in the current topic, the inquiry has demonstrated to the group that race matters, and that matters of race are "speak-able" and important to work through. If race is a factor, the therapist must show patience in allowing this reality to be seen, named and the resulting affect tolerated, titrated, and eventually transformed into faith, hope, and change.

The therapist awakens group members to the denial in the group, and vertical split within the members, when the group is invited to become conscious and aware of previously denied or disowned racism/white supremacy. In working with a group member, the therapist might say: "Might there be something about person X that brings up these feelings in you?" This split is usually articulated as "I am not a racist" with shame affect prompting the initial resistance to awareness. The group is invited then to explore the possibility of racism/white supremacy being a factor in the dynamic under examination, tolerate the feelings of shame which may emerge, and inquire whether the shame feelings are the leading edge of a previously unrecognized desire to move beyond the usual perceptions or stereotypes rooted in racism/white supremacy—the desire to restore the interpersonal bridge, and to humanize rather than stereotype the other.

The therapist may offer the metaphor of the wake, when grief and loss are anticipated as the group negotiates a new identity for itself and group members. Sitting the wake can allow the beginning of a process of integration of the loss of white privilege, the loss of white innocence, the loss of "other" inferiority, and the development of a new sense of group identity—human solidarity. And with being woke, new possibilities for true comity, community, justice, equity, inclusion, and peace. Martin Luther King Jr. once wrote: "our very survival depends upon our ability to stay awake, to adjust to new ideas, to remain vigilant and to face the challenge of change" (Eig, 2023).

Life After the Death of Racism/White Supremacy

As sleep is a metaphor for death, so being awake is a metaphor for being alive. Being awake means being available for passion. Life after the death of racism/white supremacy can mean the recovery of passion. The tragedy of racism/white supremacy has not just been the closing of the mind, but also the deadening of the body (Dyer, 2017). Life is divided into body/mind, passion/dispassion, physical prowess, or mental acuity. Things body/passion/prowess are bad; things mind/dispassion/mentation are good. The dark "other" has been the container for all things body/passion/prowess. This splitting has had dire consequences. Removing feeling and passion deprives human beings of our first language, and dangerously impairs our capacity for self-awareness and empathy. I would argue that If the splitting of racism/white supremacy can be overcome, passion may be permissible for all. It need no longer be split off and projected onto/into the dark "other," who is then marginalized, ostracized, or violently eliminated.

I make one final application of Bion's thinking. Bion (1963) uses the term "passion" to represent the experience of a group which has moved beyond Basic Assumptions. "Passion is evidence that two (or more) minds are linked" (Bion, 1963, *Elements,* p. 13) Passion is evidence of the shared emotional awareness that thinking makes possible. Billow (2003) elaborating on Bion, says "Passion involves a presence of emotion and receptivity to emotion . . ." (p. 216). Passion is fundamentally relational, expansive, extensive and enlivening, "an emotion experienced with intensity and warmth though without any suggestion of violence (Bion, 1963, *Elements,* p. 13). Passion recognizes and responds to the significance of the self and others. Passion is possible as we move beyond othering, racism/white supremacy, toward recognition and awareness, as we move from the constricted racialized false self to the reality of one common humanity.

Admittedly, overcoming racism/white supremacy, and rooting out US's root Basic Assumption, will be very challenging, and doing this work in our groups will require tremendous, sustained effort. But we who have committed to working to help people heal in groups, and help groups heal, *if we do our own work of uprooting racism/white supremacy*, have an important role to play, as therapists/group members, player coaches if you will, in helping to lead our respective groups, however large or small, toward a future worth having.

If we can guide our groups in meeting these challenges: abandon denial, recover our capacity for empathy, bear the shame of what has been done in our name though against our will, and if can accept the death of the old order racism/white supremacy—in order to allow justice and equality to live; if we can achieve this, then the other can be ally rather than alien, the self-enlarged, and the fear of replacement can become the expectation of enhancement. The fear of death/denial of death can become affirmation of life—beyond a particular life, beyond a particular group identity, beyond the narcissism of minor differences, an affirmation of life 'seeking to expand in unknown directions for unknown reasons' (Becker, 1973, p. 284). Then before being replaced, we can be together—with passion. And when that time comes to an end, yes, we each will die, our groups will die, we will be replaced, we must be replaced, it is in the given order of things. Not however, replaced by an alien other, but rather replaced by someone we recognize, someone we know, emotionally, someone just like us.

References

Allen, D. (2022). *Democracy in the time of Coronavirus.* University of Chicago Press.

Altman, N. (1995/2010). *The analyst in the inner city: Race, class, and culture through a psychoanalytic lens.* Routledge.

Anderson, C. (2016). *White rage: The unspoken truth of our racial divide.* Bloomsbury.

Badenoch, B. & Cox, P. (2010). Integrating interpersonal neurobiology with group psychotherapy. *International Journal of Group Psychotherapy, 60*(4), 462–481. https://doi.org/10.1521/ijgp.2010.60.4.462.

Baldwin, J. (1962/63, 1990/91). *The fire next time.* Vintage Books Random House.

Baron-Cohen, S. (2011). *Zero degrees of empathy.* The Penguin Group.

Becker, E. (1973). *The denial of death.* The Free Press.

Berger, A. S., & Simon, W. (1974). Black families and the Moynihan report: A research evaluation. *Social Problems, 22*(2), 145–161. https://doi.org/10.1525/sp.1974.22.2.03a00010.

Billow, R. (2003). *Relational group psychotherapy.* Jessica Kingsley Publishers.

Bion, W. (1959). *Experiences in groups.* Tavistock Publications.

Bion, W. (1977). Attention and interpretation. In *"Seven Servants: Four Works by Wilfred R. Bion,* 1977. Jason Aronson Inc.

Bion, W. (1963) Elements of Psycho-Analysis. In *"Seven Servants: Four Works by Wilfred R. Bion,* 1977. Jason Aronson Inc.

Bobo, L. D., Oliver, M. L., Johnson, J. H., & Valenzueala, A. (2000). *Prismatic metropolis: Inequality in Los Angeles.* Russell Sage Foundation.

Bonilla-Silva, E. (2006). Racism *without racists* (2nd Edition). Rowman & Littlefield Publishers Inc.

Bowser, B. P. & Hunt, R. G. (1996). *Impacts of racism on white Americans.* (2nd ed.). Sage Publications.

Brickman, C (2018). *Race in psychoanalysis.* Routledge.

Bugental, J. F. & Bugental, E. K. (1984). A fate worse than death: The fear of changing. *Psychotherapy: Theory, Research, Practice, Training, 21*(4), 543–549. https://doi.org/10.1037/h0086000.

Crenshaw, K. (1995). The Intersection of race and gender. In Crenshaw, K., Gotanda, N., Peller, G., & Thomas, K. (Eds) *Critical race theory.* The Free Press.

Democracy NOW! (2021, December 30). *Noam Chomsky on Rising Fascism in U.S., Class Warfare & the Climate Emergency* [Video]. Democracy now.org. www.democracynow.org/2021/12/30/noam_chomsky_on_rising_fascism_in.

D'Angelo, R. (2018). *White Fragility.* Beacon Press.

Douglas, F. (1852) *What to the Slave is the Fourth of July?* [Speech transcript]. National Constitution Center. https://constitutioncenter.org/the-constitution/historic-document-library/detail/frederick-douglass-what-to-the-slave-is-the-fourth-of-july-1852.

Duran, A. & Jones, S. R. (2020*). Intersectionality.* In Casey, Zachary A. (ed.). *Encyclopedia of Critical Whiteness Studies in Education* (pp. 310–320). Brill.

Dyer, R. (2017). *White.* Routledge

Eig, J. (2023). *King: A life.* Farrar, Straus & Giroux.

Eigen, M. (1985). Toward Bion's starting point: Between catastrophe and faith. *The International Journal of Psychoanalysis, 66*(pt. 3), 321–330.

Fanon, F. (1963/2021) *The Wretched of the Earth.* Grove Press.

Freud, S. (1961). *Civilization and it's discontents.* (Strachey, J. *trans.*). W.W. Norton & Co.

Gantt, S. (2020). Implications of neuroscience for group psychotherapy. In Kaklauskas, F. & Greene, L. *Core Principles of Group Psychotherapy.* Routledge.

George, S. (2022). The Lacanian subject of race: Sexuation, the drive, and racial subjectivity. In George, S. & Hook, D. *Lacan and race: Racism, identity and psychoanalytic theory.* Routledge.

Grotjahn, M. (1977). *The art and technique of analytic group therapy.* Jason Aronson.

hooks, b. (1992). Representations of whiteness in black looks: Race and representational Boston: South End Press. Cited in Dyer, R. (1997), *White.* Routledge.

Hopson, R. (1992). The role of faith in the psychotherapeutic context. *Journal of Religion and Health, 31*(2), 95–105. https://doi.org/10.1007/BF00986788.

Huling, T. (1999). Prisons as a growth industry in rural America: An exploratory discussion of the effects on young African American men in the inner cities. *The Crisis of The Young African American Male in the Inner Cities: A Consultation of the United States Commission on Civil Rights* (April 15–16), Washington, D.C. www.usccr.gov/reports/historical-publications/catalog.

Kaklauskas F. J. & Nettles, R. (2020). Towards multicultural and diversity proficiency as a group psychotherapist. In Kaklauskas, F. J. & Greene, L. R. (Eds), *Core Principles of Group Psychotherapy.* Routledge.

Kaufman, G. (1992). *Shame the power of caring* (3rd Edition). Schenkman Books, Inc.

King, R. (2018). *Mindful of race: Transforming racism from the inside out.* Sounds True.

Klein, M. (2002). *Love, guilt and reparation and other works.* The Free Press.

Kohut, H. (2009). *The analysis of the self.* University of Chicago Press.

Kovel, J. (1991). *History and spirit: An inquiry into the philosophy of liberation.* Beacon Press.

Mahler, M. (2000). *The psychological birth of the human infant.* Basic Books.

Marable, M. (2015). *How capitalism underdeveloped Black America.* Haymarket Books.

McIntosh P. (1989.) White privilege: Unpacking the invisible knapsack. *Peace and Freedom.* https://psychology.umbc.edu/wp-content/uploads/sites/57/2016/10/White-Privilege_McIntosh-1989.pdf.

Menakem, R. (2017). *My grandmother's hands: Racialized trauma and the pathway to mending our hearts and bodies.* Central Recovery Press.

Menendian, S., Gambhir, S., & Gailes, A. (2021). *The roots of structural racism project.* Othering and Belonging Institute. https://belonging.berkeley.edu/roots-structural-racism.

Mitchell, S. (1988). *Relational concepts in psychoanalysis.* Harvard University Press.

Mills, C. W. (2022). *The racial contract 25th Anniversary Edition.* Cornel University Press

Morgan, H. (2021). *The work of whiteness: A psychoanalytic perspective.* Routledge.

Morrison, T. (1992). *Playing in the dark: Whiteness and the literary imagination.* Harvard University Press.

Peck, M. S. (1985). *People of the lie.* Simon & Schuster.

Peck, M. S. (1990). *The different drum.* Cornerstone.

Roediger, D. (1991). *The Wages of whiteness.* Verso.

Rogers, C. (1961). *On becoming a person.* Houghton Mifflin.

Schofield, W. (1986). *Psychotherapy: The purchase of friendship.* Routledge. doi:10.1037/027500.

Sharpe, C. (2016). *In the wake.* Duke University Press (cited in Morgan).

Solomon, S., Greenberg, J., & Pyszczynski, T. (2015). *The worm at the core: On the role of death in life.* Random House.

Sullivan, H. (1953). *The Interpersonal theory of psychiatry.* W.W. Norton & Co.

Trimble, D. (2022). Whiteness as a disease of the soul. In Hardy, K. (Ed.), *The enduring, invisible, and ubiquitous centrality of Whiteness.* W.W. Norton & Co.

Van Bavel, J. J. & Packer, D. J. (2021). *The power of us.* Little, Brown Spark.

West, C. (1982). *Prophesy deliverance.* The Westminster Press.

Winnicott, D. W. (1965). *Maturational processes and the facilitating environment: Studies in the theory of emotional development.* Routledge.

Yalom, I. (1970). The *theory and practice of group psychotherapy* (3rd Edition). Basic Books.

Yalom, I. & Leszcz, M. (2020). The *theory and practice of group psychotherapy;* (6th Ed.). Basic Books.

Zizek, S. (2008). *Violence.* Picador.

9 Applying Insights to Training

A National Instructor Designate Training Group

Alexis D. Abernethy

National Instructor Designate (NID) Training

NID Training Overview

The American Group Psychotherapy Association (AGPA) Annual Meeting, known as AGPA Connect, offers varied experiences for participants to strengthen their group psychotherapy skills. The typical format is a one-day special institute, two-day institutes, and a three-day conference. For the two-day institutes, participants enroll in a small group experience that is either a process group or a specific interest group that is more topically focused and may be more structured. In addition to meeting the criteria to serve as a faculty member in the institutes and conferences, the leaders of the process groups must also participate in National Instructor Designate (NID) Training Groups through AGPA Connect that are typically offered every two years. Participation in this training is a prerequisite for leading an experiential process group. All leaders are assigned to lead a process group in one of the two years following their NID training group experience.

Although participants have appreciated the learning that occurred during these NID training groups, two major questions have emerged. In addition to experiencing a rich process group experience led by a skilled AGPA group therapist, would it be possible to have a greater emphasis on preparation to lead a process group? Participants have always benefited from modeling by their experienced group leader and the bond often formed with fellow instructor designates, but desire for more explicit preparation for leading a process group has been a recurring request. Second, consistent with AGPA's increased commitment to addressing DEI considerations in its governance, policies, training, and practice, the Institute Committee, the DEI Task Force, and the Executive Committee made a recommendation to revise the NID curriculum to incorporate specific training for participants to be better equipped to engage cultural dynamics in their groups. In addition to these priorities, the second most common request from institute leaders and participants was whether it would be possible to have more explicit training in addressing cultural dynamics in groups.

NID Training Goals

The first offering of this revised curriculum was conducted virtually (owing to the COVID-19 pandemic) during the 2022 AGPA Connect. Learning objectives for NID were modified from the standard learning objectives for Process Group Experiences (PGE). Learning Objectives for PGE were as follows (American Group Psychotherapy Association, 2022):

DOI: 10.4324/9781003455783-12

1. Identify the phases of group development and the leader's role in each phase.
2. Identify one's role in the group and those of others.
3. Define and apply such concepts as transference, resistance, content versus process and termination.
4. Describe key process interactions in the group.
5. Recognize leader behaviors that facilitate the group process.
6. Identify approaches to addressing termination.

The revised learning objectives for the NID training groups were as follows (American Group Psychotherapy Association, 2022):

1. Identify the phases of group development and the leader's role in each phase.
2. Identify one's most familiar and more uncomfortable roles as a leader.
3. Identify countertransferential and transferential challenges.
4. Describe key process interactions including cultural dynamics in the group.
5. Recognize leader behaviors that facilitate and inhibit the group process and working with cultural dynamics.
6. Identify approaches to addressing microaggressions, ruptures, and termination.

Only the first goals were identical. The revised second goal introduced the notion of degree of comfort and discomfort with the goal of increasing participants' awareness of their tendency to gravitate toward what was more familiar and away from potential areas of discomfort. This was framed as a common human tendency and a posture that might render leaders less attuned to cultural differences and dynamics. The third goal specifically avoided the concept of resistance and highlighted more reciprocal dynamics of transference and countertransference. This lens allowed for leaders to consider the individual member's responses, the group as a whole, and the leader's emotional responses that might contribute to group dynamics. In addition, ethnocultural (Comas-Díaz & Jacobsen, 1991) and religiocultural (Abernethy & Lancia, 1998) perspectives on transference and countertransference have been developed and provided an opportunity for explicit consideration of these responses and emotions related to cultural and religious differences and similarities. To encourage an explicit focus on race this author added the concept of racial transference and countertransference.

For the fourth goal, cultural dynamics were specifically noted as a replacement for the general term, key process interactions. Key process interactions are an important focus of leaders, but without explicit mention of cultural dynamics, leaders might be less attuned to the specific cultural dynamics that emerged. The fifth goal encouraged the leader to not only attend to behaviors that facilitated the group process, but also track leader behaviors that might inhibit the group process. This included a posture of cultural humility (Davis et al., 2013) and recognition that all leader behaviors may not be helpful. Acknowledging this reality is a critical posture for group therapists. We learn from what we do well, but we and the group also gain important learning from constructive processing and working through of our mistakes. The final goal was related to a focus on microaggressions and ruptures. This referred to leader or member behavior. Participants benefited from observing how the leader managed microaggressions and repaired ruptures.

NID Resources

In addition to a two-day experience focused on the above goals, participants received the reference list below (see Table 9.1) from which the training was derived as well as a 40-page

PowerPoint handout that presents key concepts and content covered during the training. Table 9.2 offers an overview of the four segments' time frame. Even including two time zones was a way to acknowledge the differing contexts that were present in the group. Tables 9.3–9.6 offer an overview of the training morning and afternoon segments over the two-day NID training group.

Table 9.1 References provided to NID Participants.

Abernethy, A. D. (1998). Working with racial themes in group psychotherapy. *Group, 22*(1), 1–13. doi:10.1023/A:1023025500831.

Abernethy, A. D. (2002). The power of metaphors for exploring cultural differences in groups. *Group, 26*(3), 219–231.doi:10.1023/A:1021061110951.

Abernethy, A. D. & Lancia, J. J. (1998). Religion and the psychotherapeutic relationship: Transferential and countertransferential dimensions. *Journal of Psychotherapy Practice & Research, 7*(4), 281–289.

Amodio, D. M. (2014). The neuroscience of prejudice and stereotyping. *Nature Reviews Neuroscience, 15*(10), 670–682.

Amodio, D. M. & Devine, P. G. (2006). Stereotyping and evaluation in implicit race bias: Evidence for independent constructs and unique effects on behavior. *Journal of Personality and Social Psychology, 91*, 652–661.

Amodio, D. M. & Hamilton, H. K. (2012). Intergroup anxiety effects on implicit racial evaluation and stereotyping. *Emotion, 12*(6), 1273–1280. doi:10.1037/a0029016.

Anzures, G. K., Quinn, P. C., Pascalis, O., Slater, A. M., & Lee, K. (2013). Development of own-race biases. *Visual Cognition, 21*(9/10), 1165–1182.

Comas-Díaz, L. & Jacobsen, F. M. (1991). Ethnocultural transference and countertransference in the therapeutic dyad. *American Journal of Orthopsychiatry, 61*(3), 392–402. https://doi.org/10.1037/h0

Crenshaw, K. (1993). Demarginalizing the intersection of race and sex: A Black feminist critique of antidiscrimination doctrine, feminist theory and antiracist politics. In D. K. Weisbert (Ed.), *Feminist legal theory: Foundations* (pp. 383–395). Philadelphia: Temple University Press. (Original work published 1989.)

Dalal, F. N. (1993). 'Race' and racism: An attempt to organize difference. *Group Analysis, 26*, 277–293.

Eriksson, C. & Abernethy, A. D. (2014) Integration in multicultural competence and diversity training: Engaging difference and race. *Journal of Psychology and Theology, 42*(2), 174–187.

Goff, P. A., Steele, C. M., & Davies, P. G. (2008). The space between us: Stereotype threat and distance in interracial contexts. *Journal of Personality and Social Psychology, 94*(1), 91–107. doi:10.1037/0022-3514.94.1.91.

Lefforge, N. L., Mclaughlin, S., Goates-Jones, M., & Mejia, C. (2020). A training model for addressing microaggressions in group psychotherapy. *International Journal of Group Psychotherapy, 70*(1), 1–28. https://doi.org/10.1080/00207284.2019.1680989.

Meyer, M. L., Masten, C. L., Ma, Y., Wang, C., Shi, Z., Eisenberger, N. I., & Han, S. (2013). Empathy for the social suffering of friends and strangers recruits distinct patterns of brain activation. *Social Cognitive and Affective Neuroscience, 8*(4), 446–454.

Miles, J. R., Anders, C., Kivlighan, D. M., III, & Belcher Platt, A. A. (2021). Cultural ruptures: Addressing microaggressions in group therapy. *Group Dynamics: Theory, Research, and Practice, 25*(1), 74–88.

Öhman, A. & Mineka, S. (2001). Fears, phobias, and preparedness: toward an evolved module of fear and fear learning. *Psychological Review, 108*(3), 483.

Pinderhughes, E. (1989). *Understanding race, ethnicity, and power: The key to efficacy in clinical practice*. New York, NY: Simon & Schuster.

Rudman, L. A., Ashmore, R. D., & Gary, M. L. (2001). "Unlearning" automatic biases: the malleability of implicit prejudice and stereotypes. *Journal of Personality and Social Psychology, 81*(5), 856.

Salvendy, J. T. (1999). Ethnocultural considerations in group psychotherapy. *International Journal of Group Psychotherapy, 49*(4), 429–64.

(Continued)

Table 9.1 (Continued)

Stevens, F. L. & Abernethy, A. D. (2017). Neuroscience and racism: The power of groups for overcoming implicit bias. *International Journal of Group Psychotherapy, 68*(4) 561–584. doi:10.1080/00207284.2017.1315583.

Sue, D. W., Capodilupo, C. M., Torino, G. C., Bucceri, J. M., Holder, A. M., Nadal, K. L., Esquilin, M. (2007). Racial microaggressions in everyday life: implications for clinical practice. *American Psychologist, 62*(4), 271–86. doi:10.1037/0003-066X.62.4.271.

Xu, X., Zuo, X., Wang, X., & Han, S. (2009). Do you feel my pain? Racial group membership modulates empathic neural responses. *The Journal of Neuroscience, 29*(26), 8525–8529.

Table 9.2 Overview

1. Setting the Frame for Courageous Engagement – Concepts and Key Terms -11:30 - 2:15 EST (8:30 - 11:15 PST)
   A. Addressing microaggressions, scapegoating, and ruptures - 1.5 hrs, 5 min break, 1 hr

2. Countertransference and Transference in Leadership - 4:15 - 7:00 (1:15 - 4:00)
   A. Examining interpersonal and cultural differences - 1 hr 20 mins, 10 min break, 1 hr

3. Addressing Cultural Dynamics and Ruptures - 11:30 - 2:15 (8:30-11:15)
   A. Working through microaggressions and ruptures - 1 hr 20 mins, 5 min break, 1 hr

4. Areas for Future Exploration and Ongoing Work - 4:15 - 7:00 (1:15 - 4:00)
   A. Insights Gained and Next Steps 4:20 - 5:50 (1:20 - 2:50)
   B. 10 min break
   C. Q & A - 6:00 - 6:45 (3:00 - 3:45)
   D. Evaluation - 6:45 (3:45)

Table 9.3 I. Introduction and Engagement (Formative Stage)

• Setting the Frame for Courageous Engagement – Concepts and Key Terms
   – Setting the frame and the contract including explicit language related to cultural dynamics
   – Creating agreements, norms, boundaries, and a frame for courageous engagement
   – Addressing microaggressions, scapegoating, and ruptures
   – Exploring connection as well as disconnection with leader and members

Table 9.4 II. Differentiation (Reactive Stage)

• Countertransference and Transference in Leadership
   – Examining countertransferential and transferential challenges as leaders
   – Examining interpersonal and cultural differences
   – Monitoring ruptures
   – Confronting conflict
   – Exploring dissatisfactions with the experience and leader
   – Summary of day's learning
• What are you learning that will be helpful to you as a leader?

Table 9.5 III. Norming & Performing (Mature Stage)

- Addressing Cultural Dynamics and Ruptures
  - Exploring disconnection
  - Transference to leader and each other
  - Deeper exploration of interpersonal connections
  - Role of leader, role of members
  - Repairing ruptures
  - Continued content vs. process examination

Table 9.6 IV. Closure (Termination Stage)

- Areas for Future Exploration and Ongoing Work
  - Reactions to ending including explorations of transference and countertransference
  - Review of experience (satisfactions, disappointments)
  - Review of interventions
  - Discussion of implications for NID Leadership
    o What challenges and strengths do I bring to group leadership of a culturally diverse group?
  - Questions and answers
  - Evaluations to be completed

An Updated Revision of NID Training

As displayed in the above tables, the major components of the Revised NID Training include the following: Setting the Frame for Courageous Engagement—Concepts and Key Terms; Countertransference and Transference in Leadership; Addressing Cultural Dynamics and Ruptures; and Areas for Future Exploration and Ongoing Work. The insights from this volume have most influenced the first, setting the frame, and second segments, countertransference, and transference, of this revised NID training. Insights from Chapters 2 (Addressing Power Dynamics in Systems-Centered Training Groups) and 8 (Overcoming Racism/White Supremacy) have influenced the final segments on addressing cultural dynamics and ruptures as well as areas for ongoing work.

Updating Setting the Frame for Courageous Engagement: Part 1

Key concepts that were not included in the revised training were as follows: addressing racial enactments (Chapters 1 and 2 of this volume), critiquing and adapting a theoretical frame to address racial dynamics (Chapter 2), incorporating a multicultural framework to include a wider range of cultural dimensions (Chapter 3), and engaging in an explicit discussion of the invisibility of certain cultural dimensions such as class (Chapter 4). These content areas would be important framing at the outset of training. In creating norms for the group, explicitly mentioning cultural humility as a value and opportunity for the group would be a helpful aspiration (Chapter 3).

Setting the Frame

Although adding four different content areas to a revised training might seem ambitious, this challenge might be met by linking new content to already existing content (see Table 9.2).

For example, racial enactments is a broader term that refers to "interactive sequences that embody the actualization in the clinical situation of cultural attitudes towards race and racial difference" (Leary, 2000, p. 640). Beginning with a broader term to describe racial dynamics offers a helpful, more neutral introduction that can be followed by framing micro-aggressions as a more negatively valenced interaction. Given the larger societal context, all members and the leader would be expected to engage in racial enactments, but microaggressions would be a less frequent subset of enactments.

Increasing NID participants' awareness of specific theories and intervention approaches that have been adapted or include a diversity lens are critical and serve as an important update on the revised training. Chapters 2 and 3 from this volume argue for the adoption of conceptual frameworks that include a consideration of diversity dynamics such as integrating Systems-Centered and anti-racism training or incorporating a multicultural framework to address the international backgrounds of participants, respectively. Other conceptual approaches such as Hopson's outline a deeper emotional process for participants to work through the dynamics of racism/white supremacy (Chapter 8). Depending on the training group, participants in an updated version of this training might engage a curriculum derived from one of these theoretical models. Even in this current interpersonally oriented curriculum, the acknowledgement of other theoretical models would be an important update.

A common didactic overview would also include some list of cultural dimensions, often including age, race, ethnicity, social status, gender, disability, religion, sexual orientation, indigenous heritage, national origin, and geographic location (Hays, 1996). Given the contributions of the chapter on Classism (Chapter 4), the more visible and invisible dimensions of culture could be acknowledged with a specific emphasis and elaboration of social status linking it to class as well as the three dimensions of education, income, and occupation. The leader might underscore its relative inattention in the field as well as an opportunity in this training group to attend to this important dynamic.

Creating Norms

The final update could include introducing the concept of cultural humility as a norm (See Table 9.3). As noted in Chapter 3 of this volume:

> **Cultural humility** involves ". . . openness, self-awareness, being egoless, and incorporating self-reflection and critique after willingly interacting with diverse individuals" (Foronda et al., 2016, p. 213). Being both other-oriented (i.e., curious and open) and self-reflective (critiquing, humble) serve to dismantle power-dynamics that can interfere with the cultivation of the therapist-client partnership (Foronda et al., 2016).

This posture is not only critical for the group therapist, but also for group members. In this early phase of the training group, the NID leader will highlight the importance of courageous conversations (Foster et al., N.D.) and note cultural humility as an important posture for the therapist to model and the members to develop further. The values—curiosity, openness—can be included as group agreements. The extent to which these norms are lived out by the therapist and the members throughout the process of the group would be important. In the final segment of the training potential areas of challenge and potential growth would be helpful to identify as a focus for future work.

Updating the Countertransference and Transference in Leadership: Part 2

In examining countertransferential and transferential responses, a more explicit focus on classist bias would be consistent with Chapter 4, and exploration of inter and intrareligious transference and countertransference would be consistent with Chapter 5 of this volume. This emphasis would not be to the exclusion of racial biases, for example, but it could be a rich opportunity to explore intersectional dimension of class and race as well as religion and gender. Encouraging members to consider which dimensions are more salient or more invisible in their own personal lives and their groups could be beneficial.

Building on a consideration of class and power differences and including an examination of interpersonal and cultural differences, an updated approach would include a consideration of discipline differences and potential multiple roles in the group as highlighted in Chapter 5. These roles might include associations among members not only through their work settings, but also in their connections in AGPA or past institute groups. Of particular emphasis would be the ways in which these past associations might influence them in the current training group and influence their degree of comfort or discomfort in addressing diversity dynamics. It is common that individuals may tend to avoid addressing cultural differences despite long standing professional relationships. For some, the examination of these differences may be more threatening with friends and colleagues. Exploring this dynamic in their own training group helps to prepare them for facilitating this work as an institute group leader.

Another important focus for the NID leader is to monitor ruptures in general. Chapter 7 of this volume offers a helpful reminder for the leader to track and be attentive to which ruptures may receive more attention than others. Identifying how not only the ruptures, but the repair is experienced by members of the group, is helpful. Are ruptures by all members being tracked or only ruptures that are experienced by more marginalized members? Weinberg and Gooden offer complementary as well as contrasting perspectives on how to approach diversity dynamics. Their varied perspectives are important lenses for helping leaders understand the potential range of responses of members. Groups that have the capacity to explore potentially opposing perspectives with a courageous commitment toward growth offer the healing social microcosm that will serve members in their relationships within and beyond the group. The transformational power of groups not only for individual change but societal change are powerfully exemplified in Dr. Allen's community-based groups in the Bahamas (Abernethy et al., 2018) as members choose forgiveness and repair instead of perpetuating cycles of violence.

Confronting conflict in the group is important work in this second segment. A more explicit focus on cultural dynamics typically offers more opportunity for conflicts to surface and member's sensitivity to conflict is normally heightened. In updating this revised NID training considering the insights from Chapter 8, the NID leader would be challenged to not only focus on racism, but also include the term white supremacy. For a racially homogenous group of members who have experienced racism, this might be experienced as a welcome opportunity for solidarity. For a racially heterogeneous or all white group, this would be a more challenging experience.

This update would include the leader's version of Hopson's description of white supremacy, as noted in Chapter 8. The update might begin with an acknowledgment of the pervasiveness of racial enactment. A recognition of the reality of this logically would flow toward the realization of the pervasiveness of one category of racial enactment, racism/white supremacy. This understanding, although powerful and provocative allows for a refreshing opportunity to work on rather than simply react to a corrosive dimension of our lives and relationships in our groups and beyond. The leader would prepare the group for a deeper dive that white supremacy does not only refer to the more violent scale events and encounters, but everyday interactions. Key points to emphasize would include use of some of his vivid imagery (Chapter 8): racism/white supremacy is keyed to skin color; racism/white supremacy is the larger field out of which racism emerges, and; it is the figure/ground of othering.

The NID leader might then encourage the group to consider what might facilitate and impede their ability to observe the dynamics and potential conflicts associated with white supremacy in this training group as the group attends to dynamics of power, preference, preference, and privilege in this group. Implementing Hopson's insights related to denial and impaired empathy, the group would be informed that a common response is to deny even the presence of white supremacy. The challenge associated with this is that frequently the pain associated with racism is overlooked, ignored, or disregarded. This impairs our ability to be empathic. Potential questions for this training group may include, "What would make it hard to see white supremacy in this group? What might be helpful to us in seeing it and even talking about it, even if lightly?" Hopson's emphasis on the ground of racism. In addition, deeper consideration of the intersectionality of additional oppressive systems including sexism, ableism, homophobia, etc. is critical ground as well. Useful exploration would include what oppressive dynamics are more or less visible in the group.

The next question related to the revised training outline (Table 9.4) for the group to engage would be exploring dissatisfaction with the experience and the leader. This dissatisfaction might easily include general dissatisfaction and also an opportunity to process the more explicit focus on racism/white supremacy. Members would be encouraged to reflect personally and take up the opportunity to engage this more deeply on the second day of the institute.

Updating the Addressing Cultural Dynamics and Ruptures: Part 3

This third segment of NID training is a natural opportunity to engage in more in-depth work related to connections and ruptures. The mutual commitment of the organization and the group members may help to strengthen the commitment within the group to engage in this deeper work for the good of our AGPA community and our world. This aspiration as well as the opportunity of this social microcosm would be highlighted. In the exploration of disconnection, connection, and transference, more explicit initial examination of shame would be important. Hopson describes this in Chapter 8. Others have also outlined the importance of working through shame in addressing racism (Stevens & Abernethy, 2017). Preparing the group for this work might include a discussion of the challenge and opportunity of exposure and revealing one's complicity in racism/white supremacy. The potential pain and shame might be mitigated by the shared experience of this shame as a group. Building a sense of shared experience related to shame would be critical in fostering this type of exploration in the context of an institute group:

> Shame which signals an unintended disruption in the interpersonal bridge (Kaufman, 1992) can mobilize the desire for restored human connection. This is a particularly powerful element of group therapy. If group members can bear to do the shame-work—acknowledge and work through shame, in close proximity to others, the need to continue

to deny the pervasive reality of racism/white supremacy is lessened. . . . If group members can tolerate it, shame can prompt vigilance against participation in furthering racism/white supremacy. . . . Shame, when tolerated, can provide wisdom toward restoration and repair, and can prompt a shift from allegiance to norms and ideas which objectify and create the "other," to solidarity with the human family—a necessary step in overcoming racism/white supremacy (Van Bavel & Packer, 2021).

Clearly, in a two-day institute, shame cannot be fully worked through, but if a leader is vigilant and remains attuned to this dynamic, there may be an opportunity to do some work with the group as a whole or some members that would serve as an invaluable model for group leadership.

Finally, the fear of death is related to the existential fear that underlies resisting change. Hopson describes this in Chapter 8:

> As group members engage the possibility for change in regard to racism/white supremacy, the therapist has the opportunity to hold space for the group to titrate the feelings around the reality of loss and the fear of the unfamiliar new self (or society) which may be possible. Fear of extinction through relinquishing racial group identification is named and challenged, and alternative identificatory possibilities are offered (e.g., human solidarity rather than subgroup exclusivism).

Earlier the group may be reluctant to observe white supremacy. As their denial eases and they witness how racism/white supremacy impairs their empathy and evokes shame, even as members might desire to relinquish it, there is recognition of the loss associated with its abandonment. White supremacy is such a familiar and organizing principle, who are we without it, even with its horrors?

Updating Further Exploration and Ongoing Work: Part 4

How does the group move forward after such a stark uncovering of profound and emotionally charged truths? The revised training already incorporated Ken Hardy's "muscles for cultural competence" that he shared during his Special Institute in 2020 at AGPA Connect (see Table 9.7): Intensity—moving beyond our comfort zone; intimacy—deepening connections, not simply increasing intensity; transparency—showing ourselves and being seen; congruency—being more synchronous in feeling, thinking, and behavior; and complexity—deep willingness to hear opposing positions despite your strong beliefs. Merging these insights with Hopson's chapter in this volume helps clarify a new frame for this updated training. The leader should end with this as in the revised training but should also begin with these insights as a way of framing the fourth learning objective: describe key process interactions including cultural dynamics in the group. These five dimensions (intensity, intimacy, transparency, congruency, and complexity) should be noted as process outcomes. The focus on addressing white supremacy is to move everyone beyond their comfort zone, but not for the purpose of disconnection, but for the purpose of connection. A goal is to see ourselves more fully and one another and to be more congruent in our feelings, thoughts, and behavior. Finally, to be able to contain the reality of white supremacy that includes a protective urge to exclude and harm others for survival purposes and the reality that others have been deeply hurt and marginalized by others.

Table 9.7 Ken Hardy Muscles (2022)

- Intensity – stretch beyond our comfort zone
  - Saying one thing more than comfortable
- Intimacy
  - You can increase intensity without increasing intimacy
  - Unraveling with increased intensity means that there is not intimacy
  - Escalating not fostering intimacy
- Transparency – show myself and be seen
  - Share but not be seen
  - Be seen, but not show
- Congruency
  - Everything is synchronous, in harmony, e.g., feeling, thinking, and behavior
- Complexity
  - Hold two opposing positions and value it, but profoundly disagree with it
  - Willingness to hear the other person

Ethical Implications and Conclusion

At a time in our world when an examination of cultural issues and particularly racism are hotly debated and polarizing topics, the ethical expectation for group therapists to engage cultural dynamics and their myriad connections to mental health pose a particular challenge in a typical heterogeneous or even more homogeneous therapy group as illustrated effectively in Chapter 5 in this volume. The direct examination of these issues poses an even greater challenge as therapists may be confronted on overemphasizing (as referenced in Chapter 7 of this volume) or underemphasizing these dimensions. What is clear is that many group therapists in AGPA and beyond are asking for assistance and preparation to engage these issues more fully and effectively. This chapter highlights the importance of updating and enhancing our existing tools, theories, and interventions so that we can more effectively meet the current challenges and opportunities that emerge in our groups. Connection across difference is more difficult than ever, it seems. Polarization around these differences is destroying families, churches, organizations, and relationships. Group therapy might provide a healing social microcosm that provides an opportunity for leaders and members to forge a deeper connection through this pain.

One of the ethical principles of The American Psychological Association is Justice (American Psychological Association, 2017):

> **Principle D:** Psychologists recognize that fairness and justice entitle all persons to access to and benefit from the contributions of psychology and to equal quality in the processes, procedures, and services being conducted by psychologists. Psychologists exercise reasonable judgment and take precautions to ensure that their potential biases, the boundaries of their competence, and the limitations of their expertise do not lead to or condone unjust practices.

An ethical guideline for group therapists also states (American Group Psychotherapy Association, 2002):

> 1.3 The group psychotherapist shall not practice or condone any form of discrimination that includes, but is not limited to nationality, ethnicity, race, gender, gender identity,

sexual orientation, size, disability, age, religion, socioeconomic status or cultural background, except that this guideline shall not prohibit group therapy practice with population specific or problem specific groups.

Group therapy training needs to provide enhanced opportunities for group therapists to learn how to provide healing, just, and nondiscriminatory contexts for patients to flourish. Insights from this volume offer invaluable examples of approaches that will help lead group therapy theory, practice, and training toward this goal.

References

Abernethy, A. D., Allen, D. F., & Carroll, M. A. (2018). Adapting group therapy to address real world problems: Insights from groups offered in the Bahamas. *International Journal of Group Psychotherapy, 68*(1), 17–34. https://doi.org/10.1080/00207284.2017.1335582.

Abernethy, A. D. & Lancia, J. J. (1998). Religion and the psychotherapeutic relationship: Transferential and countertransferential dimensions. *Journal of Psychotherapy Practice & Research, 7*(4), 281–289.

American Group Psychotherapy Association. (2002, February). *American Group Psychotherapy Association and International Board for Certification of Group Psychotherapists Guidelines for Ethics*. Retrieved August 1, 2023, from https://www.agpa.org/home/practice-resources/ethics-in-group-therapy.

American Group Psychotherapy Association. (2022, March). *Process Group Experience*. Retrieved August 1, 2023, from https://agpa.org/home/continuing-ed-meetings-events-training/agpa-connect-2022/2022-two-day-institute-sections/2022-process-group-experience-sections.

American Psychological Association. (2017). *Ethical principles of psychologists and code of conduct*. www.apa.org/ethics/code.

Comas-Díaz, L. & Jacobsen, F. M. (1991). Ethnocultural transference and countertransference in the therapeutic dyad. *American Journal of Orthopsychiatry, 61*(3), 392–402. https://doi.org/10.1037/h0.

Davis, D. E., Worthington, E. L., Hook, J. N., Emmons, R. A., Hill, P. C., Bollinger, R. A., & Van Tongeren, D. R. (2013). Humility and the development and repair of social bonds: Two longitudinal studies. *Self and Identity, 12*(1), 58–77. https://doi.org/10.1080/15298868.2011.636509.

D'Angelo, R. (2018). *White Fragility*. Beacon Press.

Foronda, C., MacWilliams, B., & McArthur, E. (2016). Interprofessional communication in healthcare: An integrative review. *Nurse education in practice, 19*, 36–40. https://doi.org/10.1016/j.nepr.2016.04.005.

Foster, J., Engebretson, S., Litzinger, J. (who first coined the term courageous conversation), & DeLong, W. (2005). in Courageous conversations: The teaching and learning of pastoral supervision courageous conversations about race: A field guide for achieving equity in schools, written by Glenn Singleton and Curtis Linton as part of the Pacific Educational Group.

Hays, P. A. (1996). Addressing the complexities of culture and gender in counseling. *Journal of Counseling & Development, 74*(4): 332–338. https://doi.org/10.1002/j.1556-6676.1996.tb01876.x.

Kaufman, R. (1992). The challenge of total quality management in education. *International Journal of Educational Reform, 1*(2), 149–165. https://doi.org/10.1177/105678799200100206.

Mills, C. W. (2022). *The racial contract, 25th Anniversary Edition*. Cornell University Press.

Stevens, F. L. & Abernethy, A. D. (2017). Neuroscience and racism: The power of groups for overcoming implicit bias. *International Journal of Group Psychotherapy, 68*(4) 561–584. https://doi.org/10.1080/00207284.2017.1315583.

Van Bavel, J. J. & Packer, D. J. (2021). *Harnessing our shared identities to improve performance, increase cooperation, and promote social harmony*. Little, Brown Spark.

Index